Disorders of the
Peripheral Fundus

William Tasman, M.D., F.A.C.S.

Co-Director, Retina Service
Wills Eye Hospital;
Professor of Ophthalmology
Thomas Jefferson University;
Professor and Director,
Department of Ophthalmology
Medical College of Pennsylvania;
Consultant,
Children's Hospital;
Attending Surgeon,
Chestnut Hill Hospital, Philadelphia

Jerry A. Shields, M.D., F.A.C.S.

Attending Surgeon and Director,
Oncology Unit, Wills Eye Hospital;
Associate Professor of Ophthalmology
Thomas Jefferson University;
Consultant,
Children's Hospital, Philadelphia

Disorders of the Peripheral Fundus

HARPER & ROW, PUBLISHERS

HAGERSTOWN

Cambridge
New York
Philadelphia
San Francisco

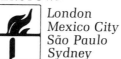

London
Mexico City
São Paulo
Sydney

1817

The authors and publisher have exerted every effort to ensure that drug selection and dosage set forth in this text are in accord with current recommendations and practice at the time of publication. However, in view of ongoing research, changes in government regulations, and the constant flow of information relating to drug therapy and drug reactions, the reader is urged to check the package insert for each drug for any change in indications and dosage and for added warnings and precautions. This is particularly important when the recommended agent is a new and/or infrequently employed drug.

80 81 82 83 84 85   10 9 8 7 6 5 4 3 2 1

Library of Congress Cataloging in Publication Data

Tasman, William
     Disorders of the peripheral fundus.

     Includes index.
       1. Fundus oculi—Diseases.   I. Shields, Jerry A.,
joint author.   II. Title.
RE545.T37   617.7'3   79-21449
ISBN 0-06-142530-3

To Alice Lea, Jim, Alice, and Graham

Contents

Foreword

I deem it a privilege to be asked to write the foreword to this book. I have known both authors since they entered the field of ophthalmology. The senior author has, for years, been interested in the retinopathy of prematurity, which probably stimulated his interest in the peripheral retina. The junior author has had a special interest in ocular pathology and now is in charge of the oncology unit of the Retina Service. This large referral service provides a wealth of material that frequently involves utilizing many modalities in arriving at a differential diagnosis. This volume is especially valuable because of its classification of diseases of the peripheral retina, a listing of the clinical features, and a brief description of the pathogenesis of the condition. The differential diagnosis and appropriate therapy is included where indicated.

Having watched the evolution of their work over the past decade, I think we are very fortunate to have the two foremost teachers on the Retina Service collaborate in writing this volume. It is obviously based on an enormous exposure to clinical material and its accurate documentation, as evidenced by the fact that most of the illustrations are original.

The authors have performed a great service to ophthalmology in presenting this material in such a comprehensive manner.

P. Robb McDonald, M.D.

Preface

The purpose of this book is to provide physicians with a handy reference dealing with diseases of the peripheral fundus. For the beginning resident, basic material on the available diagnostic modalities has been included, as well as a classification of disease entities. For the resident completing his training, this volume will provide a review of the clinical and pathologic features of peripheral fundus diseases. Finally, for the busy practitioner, this book is intended as a quick reference with photographs, so that peripheral fundus problems may be more easily identified.

The first two chapters discuss the anatomy of the peripheral fundus and methods of examination. The subsequent chapters consider the clinical and pathologic features of hereditary, developmental, inflammatory, vascular, neoplastic, degenerative, and traumatic disorders of the peripheral fundus. Many of the conditions discussed involve the posterior fundus as well as the periphery, but emphasis is placed primarily upon disease manifestations as they occur in the periphery. Disorders exclusively involving the posterior fundus are not considered.

The authors are particularly indebted to a number of individuals who have helped to make this publication possible. The clinical material utilized was made available by the ophthalmologists in Pennsylvania, New Jersey, and nearby states who customarily refer patients to the Retina Service. We are also grateful to the staff physicians of Wills Eye Hospital, especially the members of the Retina Service, who have kindly allowed us to include their patients and to take fundus photographs. The pictures were taken by or under the supervision of Mr. Terry Tomer and Mr. Donald Morozin of the Diagnostic Photography Unit of the Retina Service. Mr. David Silva processed the photographic material and Ms. Karen Albert and Ms. Laurel Cook did the art work.

Manuscript assistance and references were provided by Ms. Thea Fischer. Drs. William Richard Green, Charles Schepens, and Robert Foos were kind enough to lend us slides and we are grateful to Doctor Foos for reviewing the chapter on anatomy. Doctors William Benson and H. MacKenzie

Freeman, Ms. Linda Fried and Mrs. Alice Lea Tasman provided helpful suggestions after reviewing the manuscript and Jim Tasman did much of the photocopying. Above all, we are indebted to Mrs. Edie Rosen, Mrs. Mary Kennedy, and Ms. Thea Fischer for patiently typing and retyping the manuscript.

William Tasman, M.D.
Jerry A. Shields, M.D.

Disorders of the
Peripheral Fundus

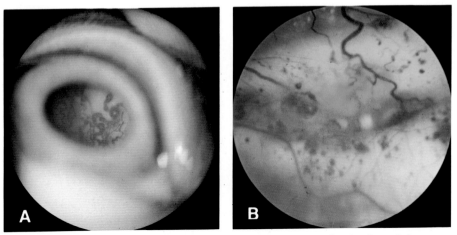

PLATE 1. *A* and *B*. Peripheral aneurysmal changes in the fundus of the periphery of two patients with retinal telangiectasia.

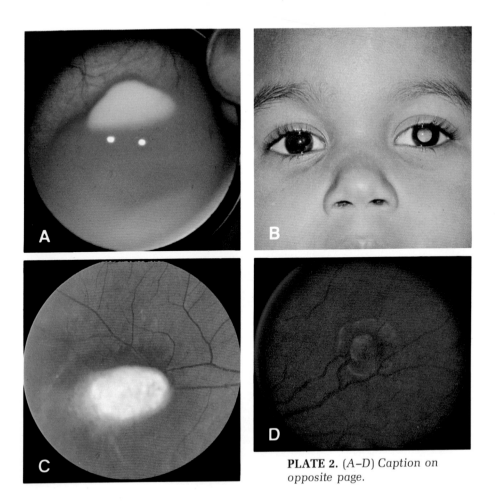

PLATE 2. *(A–D)* Caption on opposite page.

PLATE 2. *A.* Fundus photograph of a small peripheral retinoblastoma as seen by indirect ophthalmoscopy and scleral depression. *B.* Leukocoria of the left eye secondary to an advanced retinoblastoma. *C.* Fundus photograph of a calcified astrocytoma (astrocytic hamartoma) of the retina. *D.* Fundus photograph of a capillary hemangioma of the retina in a patient with von Hippel-Lindau disease.

PLATE 3. *A.* Bullous retinoschisis inferior temporally. *B.* Horseshoe retinal tear occurring in an area of lattice degeneration. *C.* Giant retinal break. *D.* Traumatic retinal detachment with superior and inferior temporal retinal dialysis.

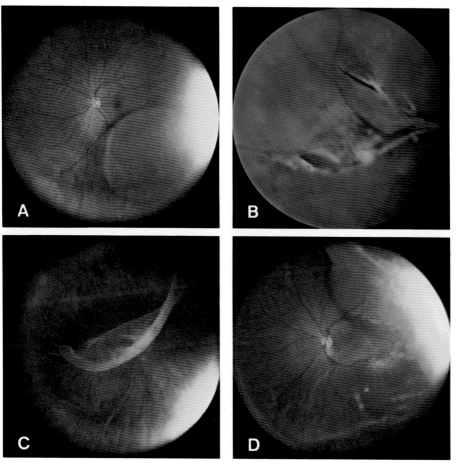

1

Anatomy of the Peripheral Fundus

In recent years, with the advent of binocular indirect ophthalmoscopy, the use of scleral depression, and biomicroscopy of the peripheral fundus, our understanding of the anatomy of the peripheral fundus has become more sophisticated. Today's residents in ophthalmology are accomplished at examining and identifying the normal and pathologic variations occurring in the peripheral retina and pars plana. With this in mind the following anatomical subdivisions of the peripheral fundus are presented in the hope of enhancing the understanding of this intriguing area of the eye.

ANATOMICAL BOUNDARIES

Equatorial and Ora Serrata Regions

The fundus may be separated into central (posterior) and peripheral (anterior) portions by a circle passing through the posterior edge of the scleral entrance of each vortex vein. In addition, the peripheral fundus may be subdivided into two areas: (1) an equatorial region about 4 disc diameters (5.83 mm.) wide, extending approximately 2 disc diameters (3 mm.) on either side of the anatomical equator; and (2) an ora serrata region, or extreme fundus periphery, a zone about 3.0 disc diameters (4.73 mm.) in width, extending on either side of the ora serrata (Figs. 1-1 and 1-2). The anatomical equator is located approximately 2 disc diameters (3 mm.) anterior to the entrance of the scleral canals. Thus, the vortex veins become important landmarks in separating the peripheral fundus from the posterior pole (Fig. 1-3).

O.S.

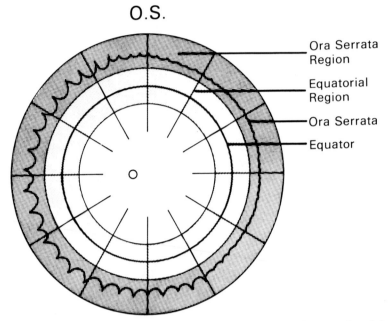

Ora Serrata Region

Equatorial Region

Ora Serrata

Equator

FIG. 1-1. The posterior pole and peripheral fundus. The peripheral fundus is divided into an ora serrata region and an equatorial region. The midpoint of the equatorial region is termed the equator.

FIG. 1-2. Ora serrata and equatorial regions. The ora serrata region is 4.73 mm in width; the equatorial region is 5.83 mm in width. The ampullae of the vortex vessels represent the posterior limit of the peripheral fundus.

O.S.

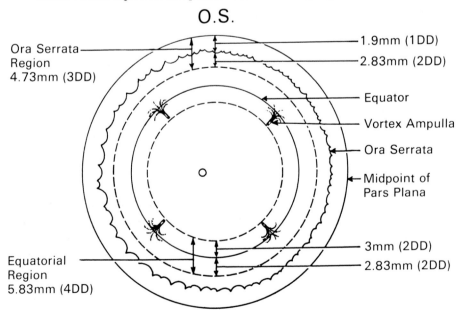

Ora Serrata Region 4.73mm (3DD)

1.9mm (1DD)

2.83mm (2DD)

Equator

Vortex Ampulla

Ora Serrata

Midpoint of Pars Plana

3mm (2DD)

2.83mm (2DD)

Equatorial Region 5.83mm (4DD)

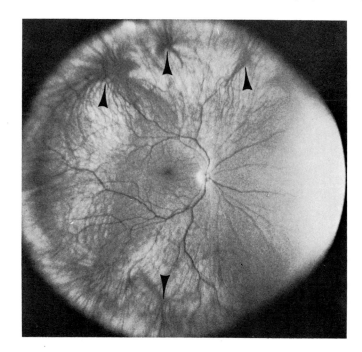

FIG. 1-3. Equator-plus (wide-angle) photograph showing vortex vessels (*arrows*) at the equator of a normal fundus.

Vortex Veins

On the basis of observations of 1478 venous drainage systems, Rutnin[8] differentiated the various types of vortex vessels which may be seen within the fundus. In some instances either the vortex veins were completely absent or all the tributaries converged directly into the scleral canal (Fig. 1-4). Other patients demonstrated tributaries emptying into vortex veins which in turn entered the scleral canal (Fig. 1-5). Still others were characterized by complete systems in which all tributaries drained into the vortex veins, which formed ampullae before entering the scleral canal (Fig. 1-6).

Horizontal and Vertical Fundus Landmarks

The fundus may also be divided by natural features into four quadrants, each of which is limited by visible narrow landmarks that run horizontally and vertically within the fundus.[8] The long ciliary nerves and arteries form the horizontal boundary nasally and temporally (Fig. 1-7). The vertical boundaries of the quadrants are made up of two poorly vascularized meridional strips which are not pigmented and have indistinct borders. These strips are most frequently located one quarter hour nasal to the six o'clock position and one quarter hour temporal to the twelve o'clock meridian. They form boundaries between two vortex systems, one belonging to the temporal and the other to the nasal quadrant. These vertical boundaries are found less often than the horizontal ones. However, at least one short ciliary artery or nerve may

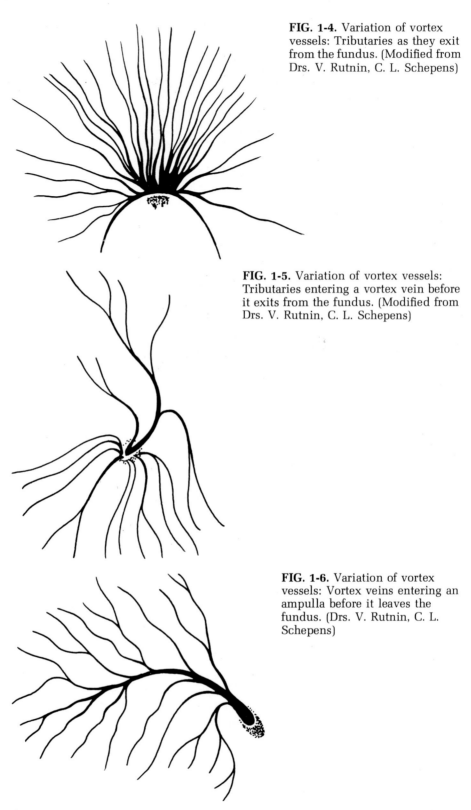

FIG. 1-4. Variation of vortex vessels: Tributaries as they exit from the fundus. (Modified from Drs. V. Rutnin, C. L. Schepens)

FIG. 1-5. Variation of vortex vessels: Tributaries entering a vortex vein before it exits from the fundus. (Modified from Drs. V. Rutnin, C. L. Schepens)

FIG. 1-6. Variation of vortex vessels: Vortex veins entering an ampulla before it leaves the fundus. (Drs. V. Rutnin, C. L. Schepens)

sometimes be noted running along the anatomical vertical meridian of the fundus (Fig. 1-7).

The long ciliary nerves originate primarily from the nasociliary nerve; the long ciliary artery stems from the posterior ciliary artery. On each side of the eye one nerve and one artery enter the sclera through separate scleral canals. In the sclera they lie close together, separated only by a thin scleral septum. The long ciliary nerve splits in two in its scleral canal, one branch being longer than the other. In the suprachoroidal space, the long ciliary artery comes to lie between the two long ciliary nerves. The artery is above the large nerve on the nasal side, below it on the temporal side, and does not branch until it reaches the ciliary muscle at or anterior to the ora serrata. The short ciliary nerves and arteries are similar in appearance to the long ciliary nerves and arteries, but are less obvious and do not accompany each other. When visible, they are near the vertical meridian and may be quite posterior.[9]

Retinal Vessels

In the peripheral fundus it is often difficult or impossible to differentiate between arteries and venules on the basis of size, color, or pattern.[9] The most practical method of identification is to trace the vessels back to the posterior fundus. The retinal arterioles and venules generally do not course together, but are evenly distributed throughout the periphery. The majority become very small and disappear before reaching a distance of ½ disc diameter from the ora serrata. The arteries disappear first, whereas venules tend to extend closer to the ora serrata.

ORA SERRATA

In the ora serrata region, the retina becomes opalescent and is often marked by small rows of cystoid cavities.[9] The underlying pigment epithelium is darker and more granular in appearance than that seen posteriorly. The sensory retina stops abruptly at the ora serrata and is continued by the nonpigmented ciliary epithelium, which appears considerably thinner than the retina. The pars plana ciliaris is more deeply pigmented than the peripheral retina and thus the choroidal pattern is obscured by that of the pigment epithelium.

The development of the ora serrata is incomplete at birth and continues in early life.[7, 12] In infants the ora serrata appears as a slightly wavy line, symmetrical all the way around the fundus and situated closest to the posterior border of the ciliary crests. During the early years of life, the pars plana ciliaris grows asymmetrically, becoming wider temporally than nasally, and the nasal ora serrata forms scallops. The concave side of each scallop is nearly always turned anteriorly. Sometimes, however, the scallops appear inverted, with a slightly concave side turned posteriorly. The teeth and bays formed by scalloping of the ora serrata become obvious at about one-half hour temporal to the twelve o'clock meridian and extend nasally to one half-hour on the nasal side of the six o'clock meridian (Fig. 1-7).

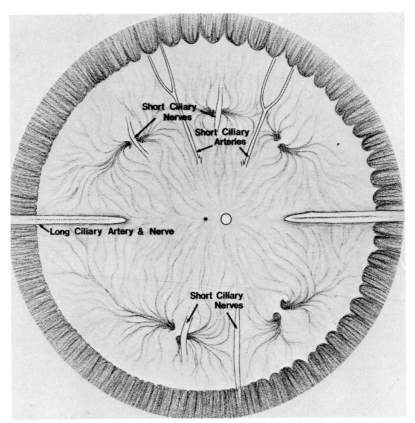

FIG. 1-7. Fundus landmarks. In the horizontal meridian the long ciliary artery and nerve are seen. In the vertical meridian the short ciliary nerves and the short ciliary arteries just to either side of the vertical meridian are important landmarks. The ora bays are much better defined on the nasal side of the ora than on the temporal side.

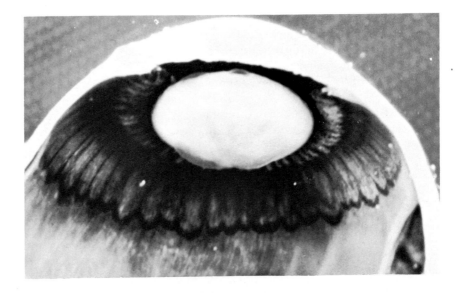

Rutnin and Schepens determined that the estimated length of the ora serrata teeth on the nasal side varies from 0.25 to 1.0 disc diameter (0.38 mm.-1.5 mm.), averaging 0.75 disc diameter (1.13 mm.) and rarely exceeding 1.5 disc diameters (2.3 mm.).[9] Straatsma, Landers, and Krieger, on the other hand, define an oral tooth as a dentate process that represents an anterior extension of the retina that projects from 0.5 to 2.5 mm. anterior to the adjacent retina on both sides.[15] On the temporal side, ora bays are replaced by wavy lines, and the ora teeth are narrow and sometimes even short or absent.

The adult appearance of the ora is reached at about 7 years of age but degenerative changes can begin near the ora serrata as early as the neonatal period. Because ora bays and teeth (or dentate processes) frequently become hard to identify temporally, the exact number of ora teeth is hard to calculate. Salzmann in 1912 identified 48 per eye,[12] while Straatsma and his co-workers noted 16 dentate processes along the average ora serrata.[16] In our experience the number varies but one is usually able to count reliably between 20 and 30 dentate processes corresponding in position to the intervals between the ciliary processes. In this regard, the teeth line up with the radial striations in the pars plana, which are also directed between the ciliary processes (Fig. 1-8).

In cross section the teeth of the ora serrata form a spur of loose tissue which projects into the vitreous cavity. Its edges are undermined and are not adherent to the ciliary epithelium. Adhesion to this epithelium exists only along the longitudinal axis of the tooth.[9]

It is essential for vitreous surgeons to know the precise location of the ora serrata. (The pars plana of the ciliary body, immediately anterior to the ora serrata, is often the site of incision for intraocular foreign body removal, vitreous aspiration, injection into the vitreous space, and pars plana vitrectomy.) The posterior border of the corneal limbus is coincident with Schwalbe's line; its relationship to the ora serrata was established in a series of measurements of 200 eyes studied topographically.[16] For all eyes studied the average anteroposterior diameter was 25.7 mm.; the vertical equatorial diameter 24.12 mm.; and the horizontal equatorial diameter 24.26 mm. The average distance from the ora serrata to Schwalbe's line was 6.14 mm. in the superior meridian, 6.20 mm. inferiorly, 5.73 mm. nasally, and 6.53 mm. temporally.[16] Thus, the surgeon has the greatest margin for error when entering the vitreous cavity from the temporal side, and least on the nasal side.

VITREOUS BASE

One of the most significant structures in the peripheral fundus is the vitreous base. It is of clinical importance because retinal breaks frequently occur along its posterior border, and, in the case of traumatic detachment, occasionally

FIG. 1-8. Scalloped appearance of the ora serrata, and the ora teeth lining up with the striae in the pars plana ciliaris. The striae are directed between the ciliary processes. (Courtesy of Dr. W. R. Green)

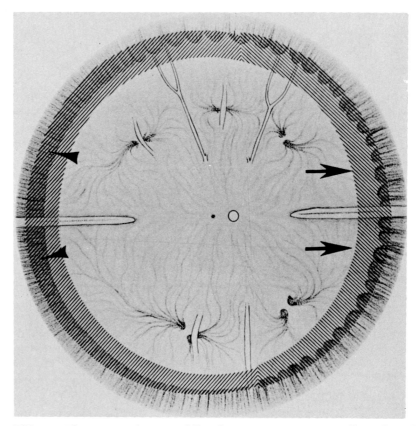

FIG. 1-9. The vitreous base straddles the ora serrata eccentrically and on the nasal side is primarily posterior to the ora serrata *(large arrows, right)*, while on the temporal side it is primarily anterior to the ora serrata *(small arrows, left)*.

along the anterior border as well.[3] The vitreous base involves the full circumference of the peripheral fundus and measures approximately 3.20 mm. in width. It extends from the ora serrata anteriorly into the pars plana for approximately 1 disc diameter (1.5 mm.); posterior to the ora it varies in width from 1.8 mm. temporally to 3 mm. nasally[5] (Figs. 1-9 and 1-10). On occasion it migrates toward the equator (Fig. 1-11).

The vitreous base represents an area in the fundus where the vitreous, sensory retina, and pigment epithelium are all firmly adherent, one to the other. It is for this reason that in some cases of traumatic detachment the vitreous base is avulsed with its underlying sensory retina and pigment epithelium, creating a retinal dialysis and a "garland" hanging down into the vitreous cavity (Fig. 1-12; see also Traumatic Retinal Dialysis, in Chap. 9). The

FIG. 1-11. Photograph of the vitreous base showing migration posteriorly →
toward the equator. The posterior border is identified by *black arrows* and the anterior border by *white arrows.* Two retinal breaks are present, the larger one being located along the posterior border of the vitreous base.

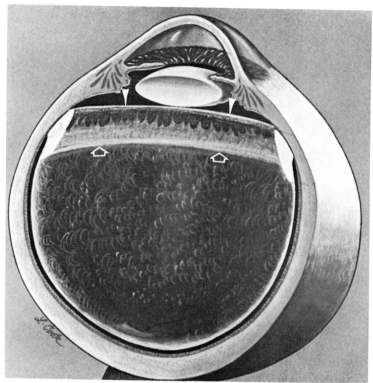

FIG. 1-10. Vitreous base is seen in cutaway section as it straddles the ora serrata. The posterior border is designated by the *hollow arrows* and the anterior border, in the pars plana, is identified by *solid arrows*.

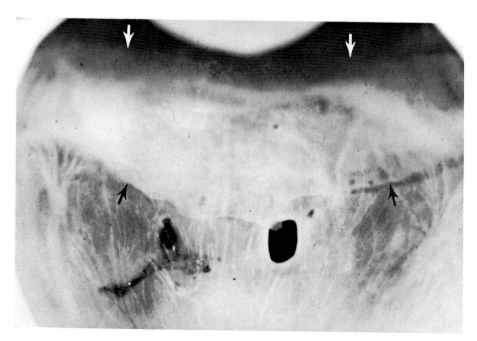

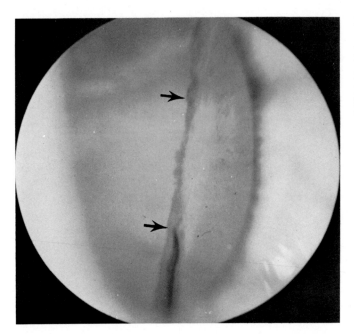

FIG. 1-12. Ribbon of vitreous base, sensory retina, and pigment epithelium (*arrow*) which has been avulsed following blunt trauma. The patient had an associated retinal detachment due to the retinal dialysis.

posterior border of the base is usually a smooth line paralleling the ora serrata, and pigmentation is subtle, if present, in contrast to the more conspicuous pigmentation of the ciliary portion of the vitreous base.

Topographical changes at the vitreoretinal juncture have been studied by Foos, who noted that the internal limiting lamina of the retina was much thinner in the area of the vitreous base than at the equator and posteriorly.[2] He found that from a thinness of 510 A. (51 nm.) at the vitreous base the internal limiting lamina thickened by 6-fold at the equator and by 37-fold in the posterior zone.

PARS PLANA

The pars plana is delineated at its posterior margin by the ora serrata. As previously mentioned, there is a firm adhesion of vitreous base, sensory retina, and retinal pigment epithelium at the ora. The sensory retina is continued into the pars plana as the nonpigmented ciliary epithelium. Cells in the nonpigmented ciliary epithelium apparently contain acid mucopolysaccharide, as shown by Zimmerman and Spencer.[18]

The vitreous base, which straddles the ora serrata, has its anterior border in the pars plana, where it parallels the configuration of the ora serrata. It is important to remember that breaks in the nonpigmented epithelium can occur along this anterior border, especially after trauma, and can, even though their location is anterior to the ora serrata, lead to rhegmatogenous retinal detachment (see Chap. 9).

Radial (or meridional) striations are present in the pars plana. They line up with the dentate processes and are directed between the ciliary processes (Fig. 1-8).

Anteriorly the pars plana is delineated by the posterior margins of the ciliary processes (Fig. 1-13). The latter are about 73 in number, compared to the fewer dentate processes at the ora serrata. Thus, the width of the pars plana from the ora serrata to the posterior border of the ciliary crests is on the average about 4 mm., while the ciliary processes themselves measure approximately 2 mm. in length (Fig. 1-14).

ANATOMICAL VARIATIONS

In conventional fundus drawing charts, the ora serrata is usually depicted as having a circumference greater than the equator; more accurately, the charts should indicate the equator larger than the ora serrata, but this is difficult in two-dimensional representations. Thus, the features of the peripheral retina and ora serrata are actually closer together than they appear in conventional diagrams.

Ora Bays and Dentate Processes

Numerous variations may occur in the peripheral fundus. For example, variations in the size and configuration of the ora bays and teeth occur frequently.[13] Deep ora bays are probably one of the most common findings, and in the majority of instances they are accompanied by variations in the dentate processes. These changes occur primarily on the nasal side near the horizontal meridian.[9]

A deep bay may be two to four times as wide and deep as the adjacent bays. Usually the dentate processes bordering a deep bay (one more than 2.5 mm. deep) are somewhat larger than adjacent teeth. Similarly, a giant tooth may occur which, except for its size, is similar to a regular tooth. Its length may extend beyond the middle of the pars plana ciliaris and in some cases it may actually touch the ciliary processes. These giant teeth are usually found in association with deep ora bays (Fig. 1-15). A tooth may also have a bifurcated tip (Fig. 1-13) or may join with another tooth to create a ring tooth, thereby enclosing a bay.[16] Large teeth and ora bays are most frequent in the superior nasal quadrant, and least frequent in the inferior temporal quadrant.

The peak incidence of dentate processes and ora bays is in the superior nasal quadrant within one clock hour of the horizontal meridian (i.e., between two and three o'clock in the right eye and nine and ten o'clock in the left eye). In an excellent study of 1000 autopsy eyes, Foos showed that enclosed ora bays were present in 4 percent of the eyes and partially enclosed bays in 0.6

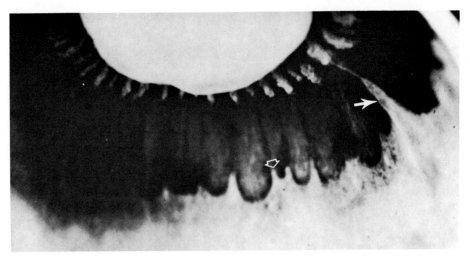

FIG. 1-13. Dentate processes aligned with the striae in the pars plana ciliaris. Note that the striae are directed between the ciliary processes. In addition a bifid ora tooth is present (*hollow arrow*) and a meridional complex extends up to one of the ciliary processes (*solid arrow*). (Courtesy of Dr. W. R. Green)

FIG. 1-14. Measurements the pars plana.

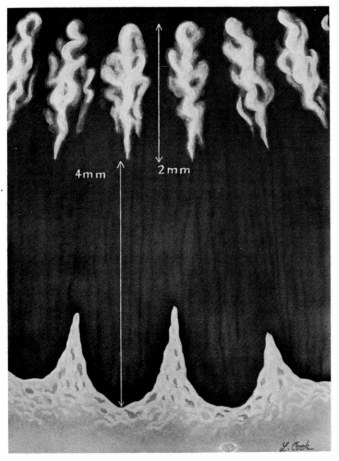

4mm

2mm

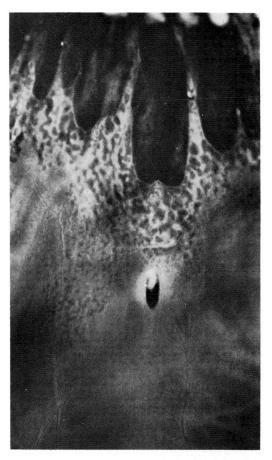

FIG. 1-15. Postoral retinal flap tear just behind a short meridional fold which in turn is related to a deep ora bay. (Courtesy of Dr. R. Foos)

percent.[2] A retinal tear was associated with 16.7 percent of either type of ora bay and occurred posterior to and meridionally aligned with such bays.

Meridional Folds (Radial Folds)

Meridional folds, usually involving all retinal layers, are another common variant noted in the peripheral fundus. These are sometimes referred to as radial folds, and we accept either terminology. However, since the term meridional seems to have more widespread use, we shall adhere primarily to that term in our discussions. As a rule such a fold begins at the ora serrata and runs posteriorly and perpendicularly to it in a meridional fashion. It is a radially aligned elevation of the peripheral retina and is often part of a meridional complex (see below). Meridional folds are found significantly more often nasally than temporally, and especially in the upper nasal quadrant.[9, 14] They have been noted to occur in 20 percent of autopsy eyes.[13]

The nature of meridional retinal folds is not entirely clear. Folds located over the teeth of the ora serrata, as well as the teeth themselves and the bays of the ora serrata, are not usually visible in the newborn. Meridional folds, when present, usually become more conspicuous with age, although Spencer et al. found that they occur equally in all age groups.[14] Bays of the ora serrata may result from a pull exerted on the retina in a posterior direction. If such is the case, then during the postnatal development of the ora serrata region, the ora teeth would form, one would think, because the retina is adherent to the pigment epithelium at the anterior extremity of the teeth. The meridional folds would then result from redundant retinal tissue caused by stretching of the retina in an anteroposterior direction.[9]

Teng and Katzin[17] have described meridional folds located at the ora serrata, most often on the nasal side, in the eyes of babies. They consider them to be a developmental anomaly, and their pictures show that these meridional folds are associated with variations in the ora bays. In their pictures, the folds were usually in the middle of an ora bay and not over an ora tooth. It is probable, therefore, that meridional folds in adults are of two different kinds: those coinciding with ora teeth and acquired after birth, and those in the middle of the ora bays and developed before birth.

Meridional Complex. Occasionally, meridional folds will extend to the posterior aspect of a ciliary process. This configuration is called a meridional complex (Fig. 1-13). The fundamental and consistent feature of a meridional complex is an atypical dentate process that aligns with a ciliary process. Both folds and meridionally aligned complexes may be the sites of small retinal breaks and require careful examination in patients with retinal detachment.

Granular Tissue

Areas of granular tissue constitute another variation in the peripheral fundus. There are several morphological types of granular tissue: patch, globule, and tag or floater, according to Rutnin and Schepens.[9] On the other hand Foos and his associates have used the term cystic retinal tuft for the larger lesions and noncystic retinal tuft for solid small varieties.[3, 15]

All types of granular tissue were found by Rutnin and Schepens,[10] most often in the posterior ora region rather than in other areas of the fundus periphery, and not seen at all in the posterior portion of the equatorial area. They again noted a significant preference for the nasal half of the globe. Within the nasal half, the upper nasal quadrant is affected significantly more often than the lower. Cystic retinal tufts, however, do not show this same predilection for the nasal area.[15]

Granular tissue is often associated with meridional folds or a retinal vessel. Granular patches also occur and appear as slightly raised plaques on the inner surface of the retina. Their borders are irregular but well outlined and they frequently have a more or less round shape. The size of these lesions varies from about ⅛ to ⅓ disc diameter (0.5 mm.). They may resemble an isolated area of cystoid degeneration.

Irregular masses of granular tissue 1/12 to 1/5 disc diameter in size may protrude at the inner surface of the retina; these have been referred to by Rutnin and Schepens[9] as granular globules and by Foos as cystic retinal tufts.[3]

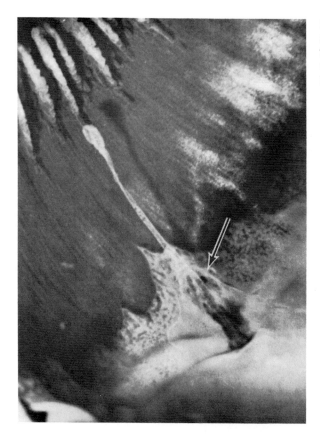

FIG. 1-16. Retinal hole (*arrow*) arising in the base of a zonular traction tuft whose thickened anterior tip almost reaches the pars plicata. (Courtesy of Dr. R. Foos)

Some globules are elongated and may be associated with degeneration and hyperpigmentation of the retina and pigment epithelium beneath and around the mass, as are cystic retinal tufts later in life. Sometimes, too, a few coarse and taut vitreous strands may be seen attached to the top of such a globule as a vitreoretinal anomaly. Such zonular traction tufts of the peripheral retina were noted by Foos[1] to emanate from ciliary processes. From there they extended to the retinal tufts where, ultimately, retinal break formation can occur (Figs. 1-16 and 1-17; see also Pathogenesis of Retinal Breaks, in Ch. 9).

Granular tags or floaters are a type of granular tissue which appear to have been modified by vitreous traction. These tags and floaters have in common the characteristic of being a definite piece of degenerative tissue which was pulled into the vitreous cavity, and retinal flap tears may occur posterior to them.

Pars Plana Cysts

Cysts of the pars plana ciliaris (see also in Chap. 8) are another variant seen in the fundus periphery.[17] These consist of a clear cystoid space between pigmented and nonpigmented epithelium located anterior to the ora serrata (Fig.

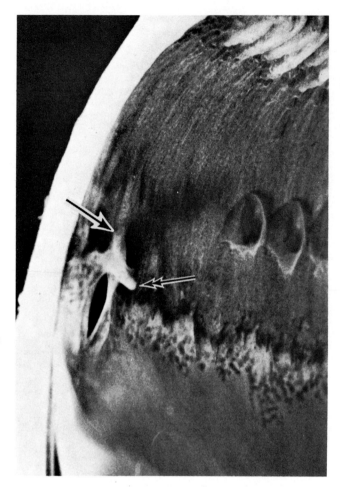

FIG. 1-17. Intrabasal (within the vitreous base) postoral retinal flap tear again associ with a zonular traction tuft. antecedent zonular traction (*arrow*) extends anteriorly fr the surface of the flap tear (*double arrow*), which is loc immediately behind the ora serrata. (Courtesy of Dr. R. F

1-18). The cysts, which have the appearance of half-inflated balloons, lie between the pars plana radiations. As a rule the overlying vitreous and its surrounding ciliary pigment epithelium remain unchanged.

Cysts of the pars plana ciliaris are believed to be caused by pulling on the ciliary epithelium by the vitreous base and zonular fibers.[4] However, no definite relationship has been established between cysts of the pars plana ciliaris and any type of eye pathology. Occasionally, however, highly myopic patients will demonstrate a marked degree of cyst formation along the entire pars plana.

Ora Serrata Pearls

Still another variant which may be noted in the fundus periphery is the ora serrata pearl (see also under Nonspecific Peripheral Chorioretinal Atrophy, in Chap. 8). This glistening opacity (Fig. 1-19), which usually forms over an ora tooth, varies from pinpoint to pinhead in size.[11] It appears in all age groups but increases significantly in incidence with advancing age.[6] Pearls are not re-

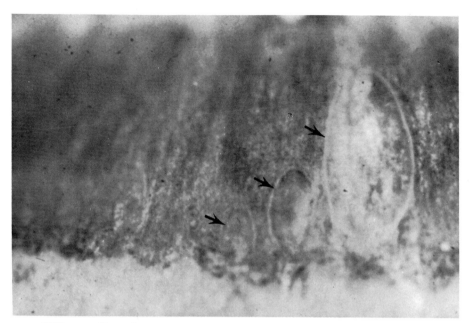

FIG. 1-18. Pars plana cysts (*arrows*) have as their posterior demarcation the ora bays and tend to lie within the striae of the pars plana. (Courtesy of Dr. W. R. Green)

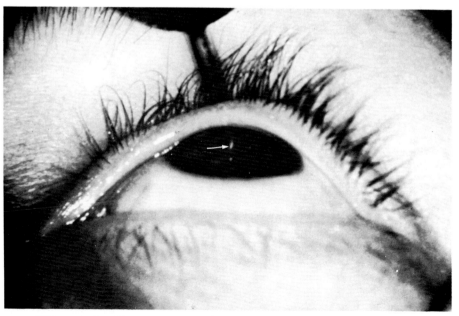

FIG. 1-19. Small ora serrata pearl (*arrow*), as seen with scleral depression.

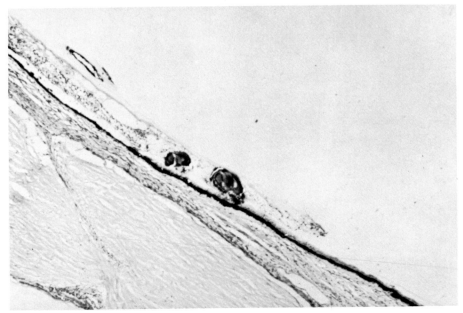

FIG. 1–20. Histologic appearance of ora serrata pearls, which can be seen to appear as hyaline-staining bodies. (Courtesy Dr. W. R. Green)

lated to other fundus pathology and are probably of developmental origin. They occur throughout the ora serrata region and are drusen structures with the staining qualities of an acid carbohydrate (Fig. 1-20).

REFERENCES

1. **Foos RY:** Zonular traction tufts of the peripheral retina in cadaver eyes. Arch Ophthalmol 82:620–632, 1969
2. **Foos RY:** Vitreoretinal juncture: topographical variations. Invest Ophthalmol II: 801–808, 1972
3. **Foos R:** Vitreous base, retinal tufts, and retinal tears: pathogenic relationships. In Pruett RC, Regan CDJ (eds): Retina Congress. New York, Appleton-Century-Crofts, 1974, pp 259–280
4. **Grignolo A, Schepens CL, Health P:** Cysts of the pars plana ciliaris. Ophthalmoscopic appearance and pathological description. Arch Ophthalmol 58:530–543, 1957
5. **Heller MD, Straatsma BR, Foos RY:** Tractional Degenerations of the Peripheral Retina. Symposium of Retina and Retinal Surgery. St. Louis, Mosby, 1969, pp 103–127
6. **Lonn LI, Smith TR:** Ora serrata pearls. Arch Ophthalmol 77:809–813, 1967
7. **Maggiore L.:** L'ora serrata nell'occhilio uman. Ann Otol Rhinol Laryngol 52:625, 1924
8. **Rutnin U:** Fundus appearance in normal eyes. I. The choroid. Am J Ophthalmol 64:821–839, 1967
9. **Rutnin U, Schepens CL:** Fundus appearance in normal eyes. II. The standard peripheral fundus and development variations. Am J Ophthalmol 64:840–852, 1967
10. **Rutnin U, Schepens CL:** Fundus appearance in normal eyes. III. Peripheral degenerations. Am J Ophthalmol 64:1040–1062, 1967
11. **Rutnin U, Schepens CL:** Fundus appearance in normal eyes. IV. Retinal breaks and other findings. Am J Ophthalmol 64:1063–1078, 1967
12. **Salzmann M:** The Anatomy and History of the Human Eyeball in the Normal State: Its Development and Senescence. Brown EVL (trans). Chicago, University of Chicago Press, 1912

13. **Spencer LM, Foos RY, Straatsma BR:** Enclosed bays of the ora serrata. Arch Ophthalmol 83:421–425, 1970

14. **Spencer LM, Foos RY, Straatsma BM:** Meridional folds, meridional complexes, and associated abnormalities of the peripheral retina. Am J Ophthalmol 70:697–714, 1970

15. **Spencer LM, Straatsma BR, Foos RY:** Tractional Degenerations of the Peripheral Retina. Symposium on the Retina and Retinal Surgery. St. Louis, Mosby, 1969, pp. 103–127

16. **Straatsma BR, Landers MB, Kreiger AE:** The ora serrata in the adult human eye. Arch Ophthalmol 80:3–20, 1968

17. **Teng CC, Katzin HM:** An anatomic study of the retina, Part I. Nonpigmented Epithelial Cell Proliferation and Hole Formation. Am J Ophthalmol 34:1237–1240, 1951

18. **Zimmerman LE, Spencer WH:** The pathologic anatomy of retinoschisis. Arch Ophthalmol 63:10–19, 1960

2

Methods of Examination

Examination of the peripheral fundus may be extremely difficult, but proficiency can be achieved with the proper equipment and diligent practice. Prior to the widespread use of indirect ophthalmoscopy, scleral depression, and the three-mirror contact lens, ophthalmologists had considerable difficulty in visualizing normal variations and pathologic processes in the peripheral fundus. Most information about the peripheral fundus came from examination of enucleated or autopsy eyes and good clinicopathologic correlations were infrequent.

In addition to indirect ophthalmoscopy, several ancillary methods are now available for obtaining clinical information about the peripheral fundus. These include indirect ophthalmoscopy, three-mirror contact lens examination, transillumination, fundus photography, fluorescein angiography, ultrasonography, electrophysiologic studies, and, in cases of suspected peripheral tumors, the radioactive phosphorus uptake test. This chapter will consider the basic aspects of these diagnostic modalities.

INDIRECT OPHTHALMOSCOPY WITH SCLERAL DEPRESSION

Although the direct ophthalmoscope has definite value, the binocular indirect ophthalmoscope has greatly enhanced the clinician's ability to detect and diagnose lesions in the peripheral fundus.

Equipment

The equipment necessary for indirect ophthalmoscopy includes the indirect ophthalmoscope, a transformer, a lens, and a scleral depressor.

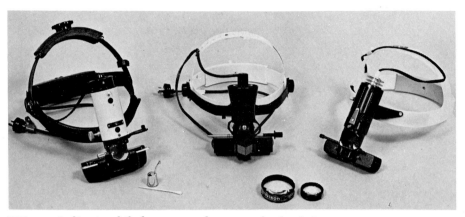

FIG. 2-1. Indirect ophthalmoscopes, lenses, and scleral depressors.

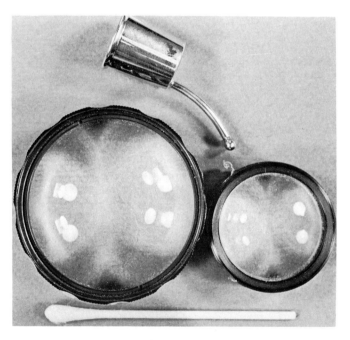

FIG. 2-2. Above. Thimble type scleral depressor. **Bel**◄ Cotton-tipped applicator for scleral depression. **Cent**◄ 20-diopter and 30-diopter lenses.

There are several commercially available indirect ophthalmoscopes (Fig. 2-1). Most are fixed on a band worn on the examiner's head, although some are manufactured in spectacle form. Several lenses are available for performing the examination (Fig. 2-2). A few years ago, most clinicians used a 30-diopter (30D) lens. More recently, the 20D aspheric lens has gained popularity because it permits greater magnification.

Special drawing paper is available for use in documenting and outlining the observations. Colored pencils and a color code are used to indicate the various normal and abnormal findings. For example, retinal veins are depicted in blue and arteries in red. Attached retina is red and detached retina is blue. Opacities in the media such as cataracts or vitreous hemorrhage are depicted in green. Conditions such as paving stone or lattice degeneration have specific designations. Lesions which are not included in this standard color code should be labeled clearly on the drawing.

Technique

The optical principles and methods of examination are well described in the literature.[4] The examination technique may vary from case to case. It is important that the patient be comfortable. Although the patient can be examined in a sitting position, the supine position is preferable. The pupils should be widely dilated with the physician's choice of mydriatic.

The indirect ophthalmoscope should fit comfortably on the examiner's head, without being too tight. The light source, the lens, and the patient's pupil should be aligned. In the examination of the peripheral fundus, a slight tilting of the lens will often enable better visualization.

One of the most important steps in this examination is the use of scleral depression. This involves the application of gentle pressure on the sclera in the region of the ora serrata, thus shifting the peripheral fundus closer to the visual axis so that it may be visualized with indirect ophthalmoscopy. There are several types of scleral depressors available (Fig. 2-2). Although some have distinct advantages over others, a simple cotton-tipped applicator will usually suffice if a commercial depressor is not available.

Advantages and Disadvantages

For examining the peripheral fundus, indirect ophthalmoscopy has definite advantages over direct ophthalmoscopy. It provides stereopsis and a wider field of view as well as better visualization in eyes with hazy media. Indirect ophthalmoscopy is especially advantageous for examining the extreme periphery of the fundus where images are often distorted with the direct method. When the technique is combined with scleral depression in a cooperative patient, one can easily examine the ora serrata and even the pars plana region.

There are certain disadvantages of indirect ophthalmoscopy. Because the image is upside down and reversed, the technique is more difficult to learn and to interpret than direct ophthalmoscopy. The necessary equipment is also more expensive. Because of the bright light source, the patient is sometimes uncomfortable during the examination. Despite some of the minor problems and disadvantages of this technique, it has greatly facilitated the ophthalmologist's ability to examine and interpret changes in the peripheral fundus.

THREE-MIRROR CONTACT LENS EXAMINATION

Equipment and Technique

Slit lamp biomicroscopy using the three-mirror contact lens is a helpful method for the evaluation of the peripheral fundus. It enables the clinician to study in greater detail lesions which have been detected with routine

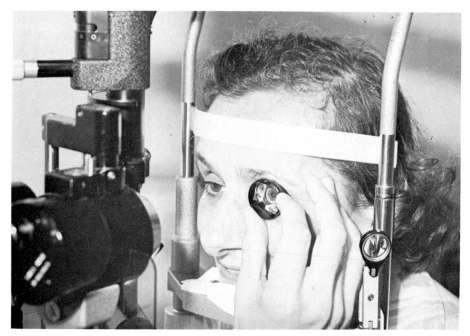

FIG. 2-3. Technique of examination with the three-mirror contact lens.

ophthalmoscopy. The basic principles and technique of examination have been well described.[8] The examination is performed under topical anesthesia at the slit lamp by placing the three-mirror contact lens on the cornea with the aid of a medium such as methylcellulose (Fig. 2-3).

Advantages and Disadvantages

The three-mirror contact lens has several advantages over indirect ophthalmoscopy. First, it provides excellent visualization of the peripheral fundus with the magnification available on the slit lamp. In addition, it can be utilized to examine the anterior chamber angle.

With the simultaneous use of scleral depression, one can obtain a much better image of lesions in the region of the ora serrata and the pars plana. The beam on the slit lamp also enables visualization of optical sections, which facilitates the interpretation of vitreous changes that might be overlooked with routine indirect ophthalmoscopy.

There are a few disadvantages of the three-mirror contact lens. It requires contact and therefore necessitates topical anesthesia. This may possibly cause corneal irritation, but it rarely causes an abrasion.

TRANSILLUMINATION

Transillumination is a useful ancillary procedure for evaluating various lesions of the peripheral fundus. It is helpful for differentiating pigmented tumors and hemorrhages, which cast a shadow, from serous detachments of the retina and choroid, which permit transmission of light.

Equipment

The transillumination system produced by the MIRA Corporation provides a bright light source and a fiberoptic system, as well as a right-angle sleeve for placing the light directly on the overlying sclera.

Technique

There are several way to transilluminate the peripheral fundus. These include the transpupillary technique, the transscleral technique, and the indirect ophthalmoscopy technique.

With the transpupillary technique, the transilluminator is placed in the conjunctival fornix under topical anesthesia. The pupil can then be directly visualized as the transilluminator is moved from quadrant to quadrant. If a dark structure such as a hemorrhage or a pigmented tumor should lie between the light source and the pupil, the usual red pupillary reflex will be absent.

The transscleral method also involves placing the light source in the fornix, but instead of observing the pupil, the physician observes the sclera on the opposite side of the eye. Pigmented tumors and hemorrhages will cast a shadow on the sclera. With this technique the size of pigmented lesions can be measured.

The third method utilizes the indirect ophthalmoscope. The transilluminator is placed in the fornix beneath the suspected lesion and the lesion is retroilluminated while the observer looks through the indirect ophthalmoscope with the light of the ophthalmoscope turned off. This is quite helpful in differentiating retinoschisis and retinal or choroidal detachments from pigmented tumors or hemorrhage in the periphery. The indirect ophthalmoscopy technique may also be used in the operating room, where it is helpful in outlining the position and course of the long ciliary vessels and vortex veins during retinal detachment surgery, and in evaluating tumors in the posterior segment at the time of the ^{32}P test, enucleation, or the insertion of a cobalt plaque.

Transillumination may also be performed with the patient seated at the silt lamp. This method is useful for evaluating lesions located in the region of the pars plicata and pars plana. By utilizing the fiberoptic transilluminator tip

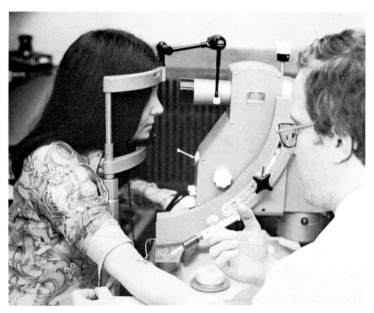

FIG. 2-4. Technique of fluorescein angiography.

as a scleral depressor, one can often differentiate cysts of the iris and ciliary epithelium from malignant melanomas. Once the fiberoptic transilluminator is placed in position over the sclera in the region of the lesion, the slit lamp is turned off and the lesion is retroilluminated while the examiner observes it through the oculars of the slit lamp.

FUNDUS PHOTOGRAPHY

Fundus photography has provided the ophthalmologist with a method for carefully evaluating lesions located in the peripheral fundus and for permanently recording their appearance.[9] A number of fundus cameras are currently on the market. Serial fundus photography is particularly useful for evaluating changes in lesions which are being followed up at periodic intervals. The recent development of wide-angle (equator-plus) fundus photography has provided a method for obtaining a better overall view of peripheral lesions which are too large to fit into the usual photographic frame.[3]

FLUORESCEIN ANGIOGRAPHY AND ANGIOSCOPY

Fluorescein angiography was introduced into ophthalmology as a diagnostic aid for a variety of fundus lesions.[9] After a solution of sodium fluorescein is injected into the antecubital vein (Fig. 2-4), the fundus is photographed, using

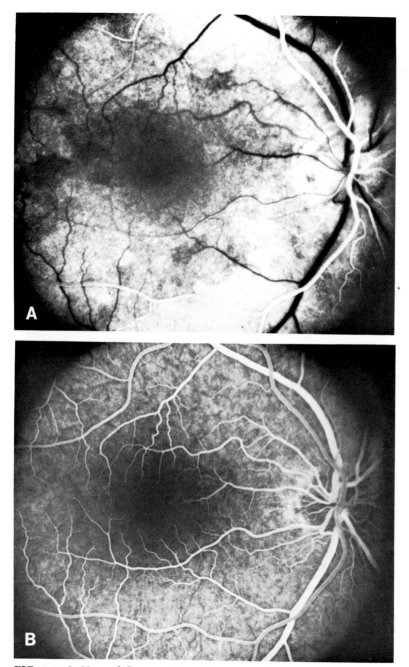

FIG. 2-5. A. Normal fluorescein angiogram in the arterial phase. Note that the retinal arteries are filled with fluorescein and there is a diffuse choroidal flush. **B.** Normal angiogram during the arteriovenous phase.

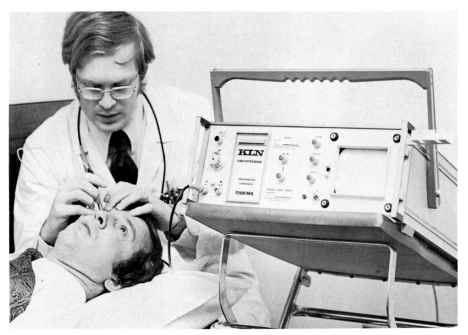

FIG. 2-6. Technique of A-scan ultrasonography using the Kretz unit.

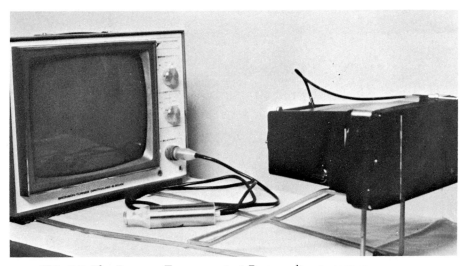

FIG. 2-7. The Bronson-Turner contact B-scan ultrasonoscope.

special filters. The angiograms (Fig. 2-5) may be helpful in making the initial diagnosis and for evaluating the response of certain lesions to therapeutic modalities.

If the lesion is located too peripherally to be photographed easily, fluorescein angioscopy may be utilized. This involves the direct visualization

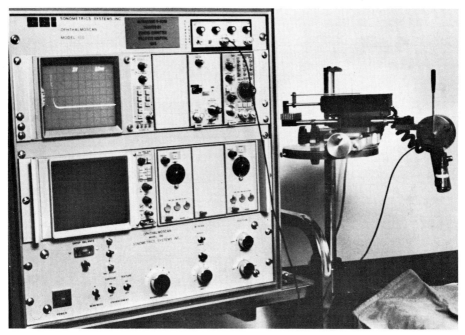

FIG. 2-8. The Sonometrics Ophthalmoscan (the Coleman unit).

of the fluorescein pattern of the lesion, using the indirect ophthalmoscope and a special blue filter. The disadvantage of fluorescein angioscopy is that it does not provide a permanent photographic record.

ULTRASONOGRAPHY

Ultrasonography is an important diagnostic technique for examination of peripheral fundus lesions.[1, 2, 6] It is particularly useful as a diagnostic adjunct in the evaluation of the eye with an opaque media, but it has other applications as well.

Equipment and Technique

A number of ultrasound units are available for ophthalmic use. Among the more popular units are the Kretz A-scan unit (Fig. 2-6),[6] the Bronson-Turner B-scan unit (Fig. 2-7),[1] and the Sonometrics Ophthalmoscan (Fig. 2-8), which incorporates both the A-scan and B-scan techniques.[2]

A-scan ultrasonography provides distinct echoes corresponding to each change in acoustic impedance within the eye and adjacent structures. Distinct spikes can be obtained that correspond to the cornea, anterior lens capsule, posterior lens, and posterior bulbar complex; diffuse echoes occur from the orbital tissues (Fig. 2-9).

The Bronson-Turner contact B-scan unit produces a two-dimensional

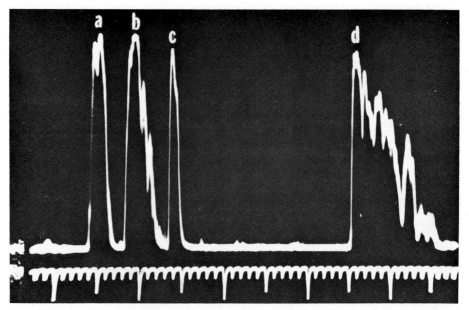

FIG. 2-9. Normal A-scan ultrasonogram. **A.** Initial spike. **B.** Anterior lens. **C.** Posterior lens. **D.** Scleral echo.

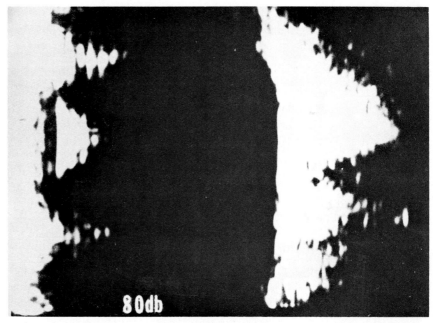

FIG. 2-10. Normal B-scan ultrasonogram done with the Bronson-Turner unit.

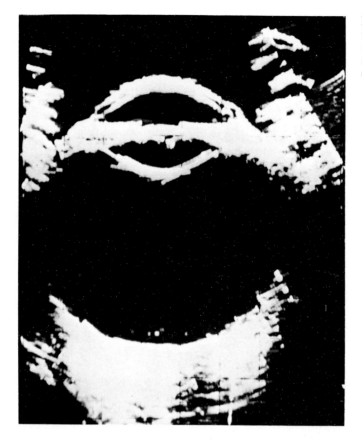

FIG. 2-11. Normal B-scan ultrasonogram using the Sonometrics unit. Note the similarity to the cross section of a normal eye.

display which resembles an anatomical cross section of the eye and orbit (Fig. 2-10). Details of the anterior segment cannot be resolved, but the posteriorly located structures can be adequately evaluated. The Bronson-Turner unit is particularly advantageous as a rapid screening test in children with opaque media.

The Sonometrics Ophthalmoscan unit at present requires a water bath, although a contact transducer has recently been developed for this instrument. This unit provides somewhat better resolution of the anterior segment and the orbit (Fig. 2-11).

Ultrasonography can provide useful information in a number of conditions. It can help in biometry—i.e., in determining whether the size of the eye is abnormal—and it can detect certain congenital abnormalities, cataracts, vitreous alterations, retinal detachments, and intraocular tumors. A discussion of the various ultrasonographic patterns as related to specific conditions will be presented in subsequent chapters.

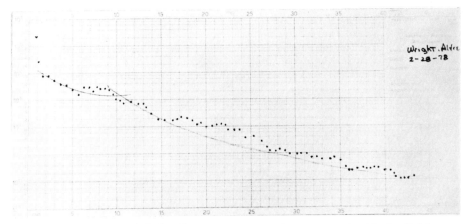

FIG. 2-12. Normal dark adaptation curve as demonstrated with the Goldmann-Weekers dark adaptometer.

FIG. 2-13. Normal electroretinogram.

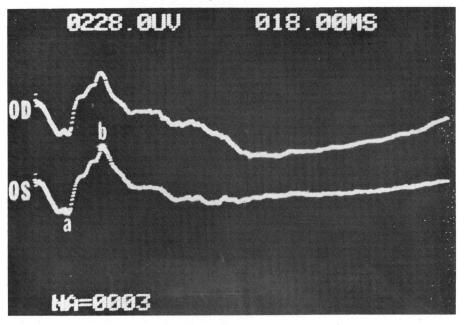

ELECTROPHYSIOLOGIC STUDIES

Several electrophysiologic studies are available for aiding in the diagnosis of certain diseases of the retina, choroid, and optic nerve. They are particularly helpful for recognizing and determining the degree of some of the hereditary disorders of the fundus. The more commonly used procedures include dark adaptometry and electroretinography. Color vision testing, more commonly used in the evaluation of macular diseases, will not be considered here.

DARK ADAPTOMETRY

Dark adaptometry is used for evaluating abnormalities of night vision and is a fairly sensitive method for recognizing decreased rod function. The Goldmann-Weekers dark adaptometer is perhaps the most widely utilized equipment. The method for performing the test is outlined in the literature.[5] A specific curve may be plotted for normal dark adaptation (Fig. 2-12). The curve may disappear in severe abnormalities of rod function.

ELECTRORETINOGRAPHY

The recording of the electrical potential generated in the retina as a response to a light flash is known as electroretinography (ERG). The technique varies with the information sought and the type of equipment used.[5]

In essence, the patient is subjected to a flash of bright light and the electrical activity is amplified and recorded (Fig. 2-13). The A wave is derived from the photoreceptors and the B wave from the bipolar cells and from Muller's cells. Abnormalities at these levels will produce abnormalities in the corresponding waves of the ERG. The ERG will be abnormal or extinguished in certain conditions, particularly night blindness disorders such as retinitis pigmentosa and related diseases of the fundus.

RADIOACTIVE PHOSPHORUS UPTAKE TEST

The radioactive phosphorus uptake test (^{32}P test; Fig. 2-14) may be used in selected cases to differentiate benign from malignant intraocular lesions.

Technique

Radioactive phosphorus may be either injected or given orally. Malignant tumor tissue will incorporate and metabolize the phosphorus to a greater extent than normal or nonmalignant tissues. The isotope ^{32}P emits β-radiation, which can be measured with a Geiger counter. The technique which is presently utilized involves the administration of a standard dose, usually 10 microcuries per kilogram of body weight.

For lesions located in the far periphery, particularly in the ciliary body region, the ^{32}P test can be performed by placing the Geiger counter probe directly over the surface of the lesion, as localized with indirect ophthalmoscopy and transillumination. If the lesion is located posterior to the equator, it often becomes necessary to incise the conjunctiva for accurate placement of the probe.

This test has been most helpful in differentiating malignant melanomas and tumors metastatic to the eye from benign lesions which simulate malignant tumors. Recent studies have shown that it is 96 to 99 percent reliable in making this differentiation. Unfortunately, the test will not differentiate melanoma from metastatic tumors.[7]

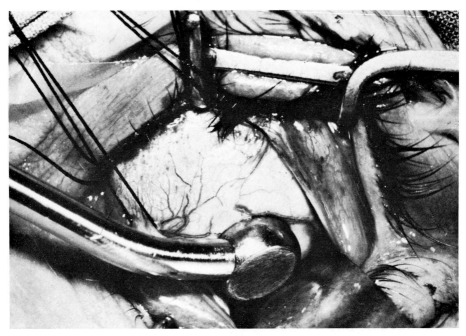

FIG. 2-14. Performance of an incisional ^{32}P test with the counting probe placed against the exposed sclera.

REFERENCES

1. **Bronson NR:** Development of a simple B-scan ultrasonoscope. Trans Am Ophthalmol Soc 70:365–408, 1972
2. **Coleman DJ, Konig WF, Katz L:** A hand operated ultrasound scan system for ophthalmic evaluation. Am J Ophthalmol 68:256–263, 1968
3. **Ducrey N, Pomerantzeff O, Schepens CL, Delori FC, Schneider J:** Clinical trials with the equator-plus camera. Am J Ophthalmol 84:840–846, 1977
4. **Havener WH, Gloeckner S:** Atlas of Diagnostic Techniques and Treatment of Retinal Detachment. St. Louis, Mosby, 1967, pp 1–40
5. **Krill AE:** Hereditary Retinal and Choroidal Diseases, Vol 1, Evaluation. Hagerstown, Harper & Row, 1972
6. **Ossoinig KC:** Clinical echo-ophthalmology. In Blodi FC (ed): Current Concepts in Ophthalmology, Vol 3. St. Louis, Mosby, 1972, pp 101–130
7. **Shields JA:** Accuracy and limitation of the ^{32}P test in the diagnosis of ocular tumors. An analysis of 500 cases. Ophthalmology 85:950–966, 1978
8. **Tolentino FI, Schepens CL, Freeman HM:** Vitreoretinal Disorders. Philadelphia, Saunders, pp 64–65, 1976
9. **Wessing A:** Fluorescein Angiography of the Retina. St. Louis, Mosby, 1969

3

Hereditary Disorders

CLASSIFICATION OF INHERITED DISORDERS

Some hereditary disorders affect the peripheral fundus as well as the posterior pole, although the posterior pole seems to be a more common site for this group of diseases. In this chapter discussion of these disorders will be based on mode of inheritance, as presently understood, beginning with X-linked recessive conditions, then continuing with those that are autosomal dominant and then autosomal recessive. Finally, we shall discuss retinitis pigmentosa, which may be inherited by all three modes of inheritance. In many ways this is an imperfect method of classifying disease, since environmental factors undoubtedly play a role in genetic disease as well. Both genetics and environment influence the development of the phenotype and hence the clinical characteristics of the disease. As an example, diabetes is known to have a strong familial incidence, suggesting a genetic influence. However, Jews from Yemen had virtually no diabetes until they emigrated to Israel, where they now develop the disease at a rate close to that of other Israelis.[3] Here urban living and overnutrition may be interpreted as environmental influences on the development of the disease.

In addition, the phenomena of penetrance and variable expressivity are features of genetic disease which illustrate the modification of major gene expression by other factors. Penetrance is an all-or-none characteristic. Clinically, the trait in question may be either visible or not visible or, in other words, it may be penetrant or nonpenetrant. But penetrance can not always be determined by clinical examination alone. A good example is provided by Best's vitelliform degeneration, in which about three-fourths of individuals

35

who inherit the gene demonstrate clinical evidence of the disorder. However, electro-oculography detects nearly all carriers of the gene, indicating that the penetrance is higher than is at first apparent. Detection of penetrance thus depends in large part on our capability to demonstrate the presence of the trait.

Similarly, variable expressivity is a feature of genetic disease, especially of autosomal dominant disorders. Thus, in Best's disease findings may range from normal fundi, through the typical "egg yolk" appearance, to multiple lesions remote from the macula. Pleotropism, or multiple effects of the gene, are demonstrated in the same disorder by the frequently associated findings of hypermetropia and esotropia. In addition, Cross has pointed out that genetic mutations which become manifest with a single "dose" (i.e., autosomal dominant traits) have a higher incidence of incomplete penetrance and cause a defect in a structural protein, while recessive inheritance patterns (causing mutations that are evident only with a double dose) produce an enzymatic defect resulting in an inborn error of metabolism.[4]

X-LINKED RECESSIVE DISORDERS

In the most common situation in X-linked recessive inheritance, a gene is carried on the X chromosome. Affected individuals pass the trait on to all of their daughters, since it is on the X chromosome, and the daughters all become carriers (Fig. 3-1). None of the sons are affected. Each carrier daughter, however, has a 50 percent chance that each one of her sons will have the disease and a 50 percent chance that each of her daughters will be a carrier (Fig. 3-2).

Stated another way, each affected male will have no affected male offspring, but runs a 50 percent risk that each of his grandsons will have the disease, and he knows for certain that all of his daughters are carriers.

X-LINKED RETINOSCHISIS

This notable condition is characterized by splitting of the retina into an inner and outer layer. Yanoff, Rahn, and Zimmerman[21] in 1968 pointed out that the splitting occurs in the nerve fiber layer.

Diagnosis is usually made at age 10 years. The most frequent presenting symptom is poor vision in one or both eyes. Probably the next most frequent is vitreous hemorrhage, while other abnormalities which lead to the diagnosis are heterotropia, nystagmus, and a known history of x-linked retinoschisis.[8]

Fundus Characteristics

The most characteristic ophthalmoscopic finding, which is present in about 50 percent of patients, is a ballooning elevation of the inner layer of the retinoschisis with dehiscence of the nerve fiber layer. This elevation, or bulla,

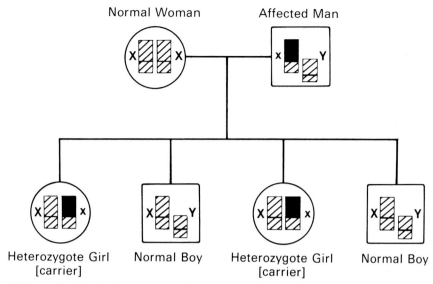

FIG. 3-1. In X-linked recessive inheritance the affected male has daughters who are carriers.

FIG. 3-2. The carrier daughter of a man with an X-linked recessive condition can expect that each of her sons will have a 50 percent chance of having the disease, and each of her daughters a 50 percent chance of being a carrier.

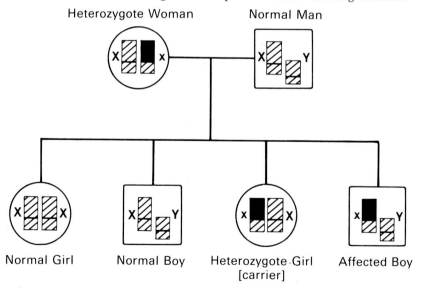

is usually located inferiorly, with the inferotemporal quadrant being the most frequently involved site. The inner layer is usually very thin and can be identified by the presence of blood vessels (Fig. 3-3). The anterior limit of the retinoschisis seldom extends to the ora serrata, while the posterior limit is usually convex and is often present as far posteriorly as the optic nerve. In

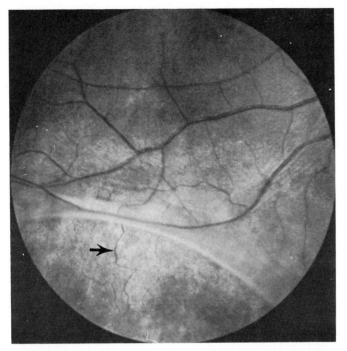

FIG. 3-3. Nerve fiber layer dehiscence. One blood vessel runs along the margin of inner layer, while a second (*arrow*) is deeper and runs toward the outer layer.

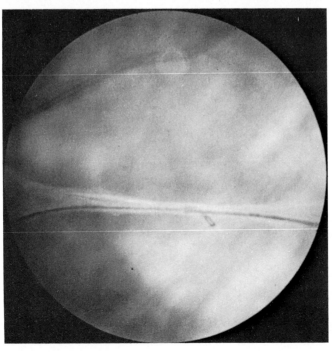

FIG. 3-4. Nerve fiber layer dehiscences in a patient with X-linked retinoschisis. Unsupported retinal vessels are a cause of vitreous hemorrhage in approximately 50 percent of patients.

some eyes inner layer breaks are so large that only remnants of the inner layer remain; these may be reduced to shreds of tissue along preserved blood vessels (Fig. 3-4).

The outer layer of the retinoschisis may have a gray, translucent appearance overlying the choroidal vasculature. Outer layer breaks are infrequent, but when they occur tend to be smaller than those found in the inner layer. Usually they are located near the posterior edge of the retinoschisis. Most often the outer layer breaks are round. Coincident with these findings one may find a decrease in the B wave when an electroretinogram (ERG) is done.

Retinoschisis is a variable condition and, therefore, may demonstrate the peripheral inner layer dehiscences in only 50 percent of cases. In addition, of those patients with peripheral changes about one-half will have recurrent vitreous hemorrhages because of the unsupported vessels (Fig. 3-4). The one constant feature of the disease, however, is the macular change. Most commonly the macula has a stellate, cystic appearance which probably represents a schisis (Fig. 3-5). Fluorescein angiography of the macula at this stage of the disease appears normal. However, as the patient matures into his twenties, the typical star-shaped cystic appearance in the macula disappears and is replaced by a nonspecific type of macular degeneration (Fig. 3-6). At this stage, without a known family history or the finding of inner layer dehiscences in the fundus periphery, it becomes more difficult to identify the condition as X-linked retinoschisis.

Natural History

X-linked retinoschisis is usually stationary or very slowly progressive. The most important manifestation of progressive disease is an increase in the extent or the height of the retinoschisis bulla. In some long-standing cases, the holes in the inner layer may coalesce or become so large that, except for shreds of tissue along the vessels, the inner layer is practically missing. It is important to realize that the progression of retinoschisis may be followed by spontaneous partial regression since collapse of the retinoschisis bulla can also occasionally occur.

Differential Diagnosis

The differential diagnosis of X-linked retinoschisis (Table 3-1) includes (1) retinal detachment, (2) persistent posterior hyperplastic primary vitreous, (3) Wagner's hyaloid retinal (vitreoretinal) degeneration, (4) Stickler's hereditary progressive arthro-ophthalmopathy, and (5) Goldmann-Favré disease. Wagner's disease, Stickler's syndrome, and Goldmann-Favré disease are outlined in Table 3-1 and are discussed more fully later in this chapter. Retinal detachment (see Chap. 9) may be differentiated from X-linked retinoschisis in that the latter always occurs bilaterally and usually shows the macular changes already described. In addition, a retinal detachment, unlike X-linked retinoschisis, most often extends to the ora serrata.

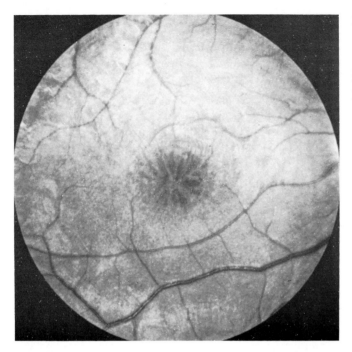

FIG. 3-5. Typical cartwhe or spoke-wheel stellate appearance of the macula patient with X-linked retinoschisis. This most likely represents a schisis within the macular area.

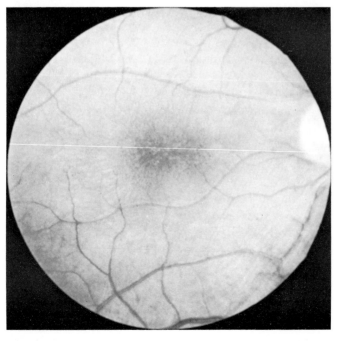

FIG. 3-6. X-linked retinoschisis after the age 20 years. The macular appearance becomes mor nonspecific, and periphe changes or a family histor the disease are necessary establish the diagnosis.

TABLE 3-1
Differential Diagnosis of Certain Hereditary Fundus Disorders

Characteristics	X-Linked Retinoschisis	Wagner's Disease	Stickler's Syndrome	Goldmann-Favré Disease
Inheritance	X-linked	Autosomal dominant	Autosomal dominant	Autosomal recessive
Myopia	—	Minus 4D	Minus 16D	—
Hyperopia	+	—	—	—
Retinal detachment	Rare	—	Common	Common
Cataract	—	+	+	+
Arthropathy	—	—	+	—
Cleft palate	—	—	+	—
Optically empty vitreous cavity	—	+	+	—
Membranes	—	+	+	+
Peripheral schisis	Splits at nerve fiber layer	—	—	+
Perivascular pigmentation (radial lattice)	—	+	+	+
Night blindness (R.P.)	—	—	—	+
Nerve fiber layer breaks	50% of cases	—	—	—
Macular change	Schisis (spoke wheel)	—	—	Schisis
Vitreous hemorrhage	25% of cases	—	—	—
Optic atrophy	—	+	—	+

+ = Present; − = absent; D = diopters; R.P. = retinitis pigmentosa.

Persistent posterior hyperplastic primary vitreous (see also in Chap. 4) is unilateral 90 percent of the time and is neither familial nor hereditary except in Norrie's disease. In the latter condition, which is inherited as an X-linked recessive disorder, there is associated mental retardation, deafness, and usually early death. In persistent hyperplastic primary vitreous extensive hyaloid remnants adherent to the disc in the inferior retina may contract, causing an inferior retinal detachment with or without visible retinal breaks.

CHOROIDEREMIA

Choroideremia is another disease which is inherited as an X-linked recessive trait and affects only males. (The carrier mother, however, may show some pigmentary changes of the peripheral fundus, though she has a physiologically normal retina.) Boys with this disease begin to notice difficulty with night blindness, often in the first decade of life or shortly thereafter. Examination reveals atrophy of the choriocapillaris and pigment epithelium, usually beginning in the periphery (Fig. 3-7). As a result, patients maintain good central vision until later life, but become severely disabled because of the loss of peripheral field secondary to degeneration of the photoreceptors. The clinical course is unfortunately a progressive one and the ERG is usually flat.[2]

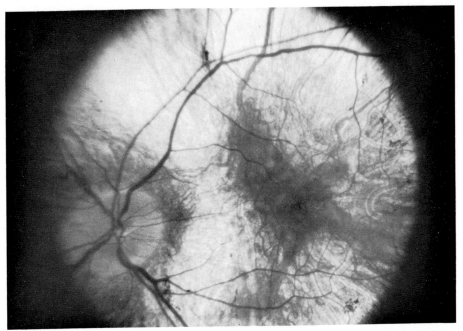

FIG. 3-7. Choroideremia in a 21-year-old male. The retinal pigment epithelium and choriocapillaris are gone and only large choroidal vessels can be noted. The macula is preserved until the end stage of the disease.

Differential Diagnosis

The most common condition to be considered in the differential diagnosis of choroideremia is ocular albinism, a condition usually inherited as an X-linked recessive trait. Recently, however, autosomal recessive pedigrees have also been reported.[15a] In X-linked ocular albinism, the eye is deficient in pigment and there is subnormal visual acuity, translucent iridis, congenital nystagmus, photophobia, hypopigmentation of the fundus with hypoplasia of the fovea, and a high incidence of strabismus. The ERG, however, remains normal, which can be a helpful differential diagnostic test in separating this disorder from choroideremia.

Persons with generalized albinism demonstrate an autosomal recessive mode of inheritance, and because of their overall lack of body pigment are easily differentiated from choroideremia patients.

AUTOSOMAL DOMINANT DISORDERS

Several ocular conditions can be inherited as purely dominant traits. For a condition to be established as autosomal dominant it should be documented through three successive generations. Males and females are equally affected, and approximately 50 percent of the offspring of a person with the disease will

Affected Heterozygote   Normal Homozygote

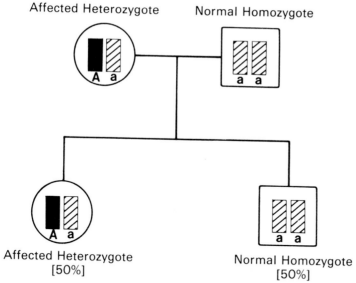

Affected Heterozygote   Normal Homozygote
     [50%]   [50%]

FIG. 3-8. Autosomal dominant inheritance. To be established the pattern should be documented in three successive generations. In this mode of inheritance each offspring of an affected individual has approximately a 50 percent chance of being affected with the disease.

manifest the condition. Stated another way, each child of a man or woman with the disorder has a 50 percent chance of having the disorder (Fig. 3-8).

WAGNER'S HYALOID RETINAL DEGENERATION AND STICKLER'S SYNDROME

Wagner's disease (Table 3-1), first described in 1938,[18] affects the entire fundus without a predilection for the lower half. It is characterized by an optically empty vitreous cavity due to liquefaction of the vitreous, and by avascular vitreous preretinal membranes, usually without holes, which may cause traction on the retina. Pigmentation along retinal vessels and sheathing of vessels are also seen but the ERG is normal. The macula is also normal. Cataracts are a prominent feature of Wagner's disease and frequently obscure the fundus periphery. In a large series reported by Jansen,[11] the malignant nature of retinal detachment in this condition was emphasized, but many of these patients may have had Stickler's syndrome instead.

Actually, most of the cases referred to as the hyaloid retinal (or vitreoretinal) degeneration of Wagner fall more appropriately into the category of Stickler's syndrome (Table 3-1). In his original paper Wagner described a majority of patients with myopia of less than 4 diopters, optically empty vitreous cavities, and pigmentary changes in the retina. None of his patients had retinal detachment.[18] Subsequently Jansen enlarged on Wagner's description and noted retinal detachment as a feature of the disease.[11]

In 1965 Stickler et al. described a hereditary progressive arthro-ophthalmopathy with an autosomal dominant inheritance, high myopia, optically empty vitreous cavities, preretinal membranes (Fig. 3-9), pigmentary changes in the fundus, cataracts, and a malignant form of retinal detachment.[17] Opitz in 1972 designated Stickler's syndrome as the most common disorder associated with high myopia and retinal detachment.[15b] Systemic findings include flattened facies, skeletal dysplasia, cleft palate, and, rarely, mental retardation.

From the ophthalmologist's standpoint, it is important to remember that in each of these entities, if the retina is detached, breaks may occur near the insertion of vitreous membranes (Fig. 3-10) which makes the prognosis for successful repair of the retina quite guarded. For this reason, if retinal breaks can be identified before the retina detaches, it is important to treat them prophylactically as insurance for preservation of vision and, one hopes, for prevention of later retinal detachment.

DRUSEN

Large drusen are frequently noted bilaterally in the posterior pole, often at a young age. Occurring as hyalinized bodies involving Bruchs membrane and the retinal pigment epithelium, they are probably inherited as an autosomal dominant trait, and occur more frequently in women than men.[9] Less commonly recognized is the fact that drusen can also occur in the fundus periphery (Fig. 3-11; see also Nonspecific Peripheral Chorioretinal Atrophy, Chap. 8). In that location, they rarely cause difficulty, although eccentric disciform degeneration may develop.

AUTOSOMAL RECESSIVE DISORDERS

In conditions which are autosomal recessive, both males and females are affected. Even when both parents appear normal, they must both carry the trait for the disease if it has occurred in their children. There may or may not be a known history of consanguinity, but the incidence of a recessive disorder is 20 times higher when such a history is present. An individual who has a recessive disease and whose marriage partner does not carry the trait can assume that their offspring will not be affected, although there is a 100 percent chance that all children will be carriers (Fig. 3-12). Similarly, if two normal parents both carry the same recessive gene there is a 25 percent chance that each child will be affected (Fig. 3-13).

LEBER'S CONGENITAL AMAUROSIS

Leber's congenital amaurosis develops shortly after birth and leads to severe visual impairment. Ophthalmoscopically, the fundus may assume different appearances. At first it may appear essentially normal, in which case the diagnosis is determined primarily by use of the ERG, which shows greatly reduced or absent photopic and scotopic responses, proving the presence of

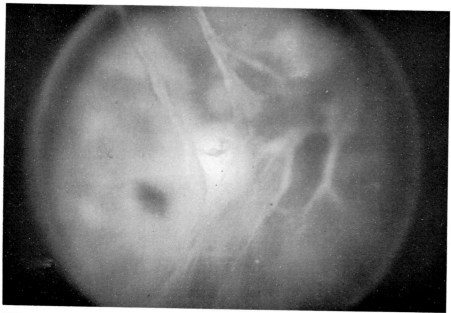

FIG. 3-9. Numerous vitreous membranes overlying the optic nerve head in a patient with Stickler's syndrome.

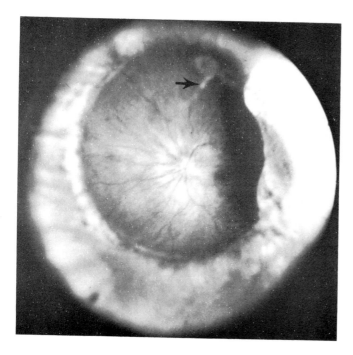

FIG. 3-10. Equator-plus photograph of a patient with Stickler's syndrome after vitrectomy and retinal repair. A residual membrane (*arrow*) can be seen.

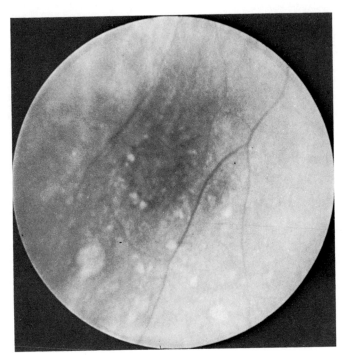

FIG. 3-11. Peripheral drusen in a 60-year-old woman.

FIG. 3-12. Autosomal recessive inheritance. In the case where one parent has the disease, each of the offspring will be carriers of the disease but will be phenotypically normal.

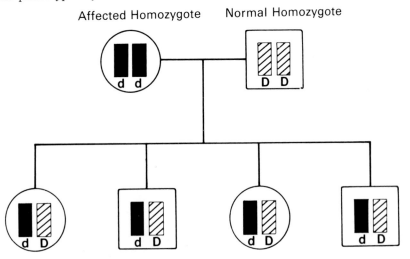

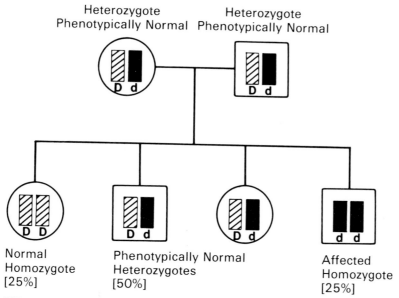

Heterozygote Phenotypically Normal   **Heterozygote Phenotypically Normal**

Normal Homozygote [25%]

Phenotypically Normal Heterozygotes [50%]

Affected Homozygote [25%]

FIG. 3-13. Autosomal recessive inheritance. In the case where each parent appears phenotypically normal but carries the trait for the disorder, each offspring will have approximately a 25 percent chance of having the disease and a 50 percent chance of being a carrier but phenotypically normal.

widespread retinal dysfunction. In other cases, pigmentary changes occur both in the periphery and in the posterior pole, giving a salt-and-pepper appearance. In the periphery they may occur as a "bone spicule," or "bone corpuscle," type of pigmentation similar to that seen in retinitis pigmentosa. In other patients, the condition is characterized by choroidal sclerosis.

Keratoconus and cataracts are often associated with Leber's amaurosis, and a particular characteristic of patients with this affliction is the oculodigital reflex, which consists of excessive rubbing of the eyes, probably with the production of phosphenes.

Leber's congenital amaurosis may be confused with Leber's hereditary optic atrophy, which primarily affects males and presents at a later age. The latter condition, which starts as an optic neuritis, is hereditary, but the inheritance pattern does not follow mendelian principles. Males are predominantly affected. The heterozygous female transmits the trait to sons and the carrier state to daughters. There is no genotypic difference between a female carrier and a manifestly affected woman. Finally, all daughters (not the expected 50%) of carriers are themselves carriers. In mild cases, visual evoked response (VER) testing is helpful in establishing the diagnosis of families known to have males affected with the disease. Steroids have little or no value.

GOLDMANN-FAVRÉ DISEASE

Goldmann-Favré disease (Table 3-1) is inherited as an autosomal recessive trait and therefore affects males and females equally. It is characterized by night blindness that is due to fundus changes typical of retinitis pigmentosa (Fig. 3-14). The ERG is usually flat. Once again, the vitreous is liquefied and contains preretinal membranes (Fig. 3-15). Macular and peripheral retinoschisis and retinal detachment occur. As with Wagner's disease and Stickler's syndrome, cataracts are a frequent feature of the disorder. Retinal detachment has a poor prognosis for successful repair, so prophylactic repair of asymptomatic breaks without detachment is indicated, just as it is in Stickler's syndrome.

FUNDUS FLAVIMACULATUS

This disease is characterized by yellow pisciform lesions located in the retinal pigment epithelium (Figs. 3-16 and 3-17). Stargardt,[16] in his original description in 1909 of juvenile macular degeneration of an autosomal recessive type, noted that many of his patients have what we now know to be fundus flavimaculatus as an associated finding.[12] Franceschetti[7] in 1965 found that approximately one-half of his patients also had macular changes in association with the fundus flavimaculatus.

The electroretinogram in fundus flavimaculatus is normal, but the electro-oculogram is altered. The condition is usually not progressive and only affects vision if one of the flecks happens to be located directly in the foveola.

Fundus flavimaculatus must be differentiated from retinitis punctata albescens (see below), which is a progressive condition that often leads to night blindness, as does retinitis pigmentosa. A helpful differential point is that the lesions in fundus flavimaculatus are, as mentioned, pisciform in shape (Figs. 3-16 and 3-17). Secondly, the lesions do not extend beyond the equator. In addition, it is uncommon for the area of the fundus just temporal to the optic nerve head to show fundus flavimaculatus lesions, which is not the case for drusen and retinitis punctata albescens.

Fundus flavimaculatus lesions may show transmission of fluorescein in some areas and obscuration of fluorescence in others (Fig. 3-17). This variation may be due to the age of the particular lesion and, according to Klien and Krill, represents an accumulation of acid mucopolysaccharide in the retinal pigment epithelial cells.[12a] More recently, Lucier and Eagle have identified the substance as lipofucin.[13a]

RETINITIS PUNCTATA ALBESCENS

Retinitis punctata albescens is a rare autosomal recessive disorder characterized by white retinal spots and often by later pigmentary retinal changes as well. Visual fields are constricted and the ERG is extinguished. Central visual acuity is also usually decreased in this condition. Fundus albipunctata may simulate early cases of retinitis punctata albescens, but albipunctata is usually nonprogressive (Figs. 3-18 and 3-19).

(Text continues on page 52)

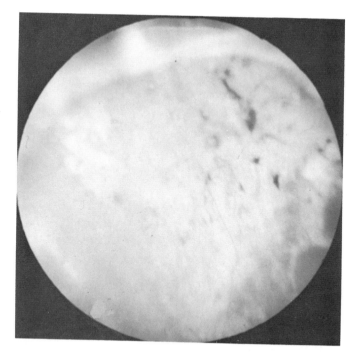

FIG. 3-14. Pigmentary changes in the fundus of a patient with Goldmann-Favré disease. Changes are similar to those seen in retinitis pigmentosa and lead to night blindness and a decrease in the ERG.

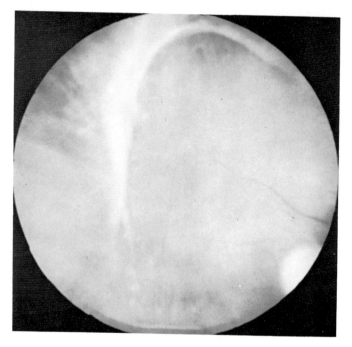

FIG. 3-15. Vitreous membranes in a patient with Goldmann-Favré disease. These membranes predispose to retinal break formation and retinal detachment.

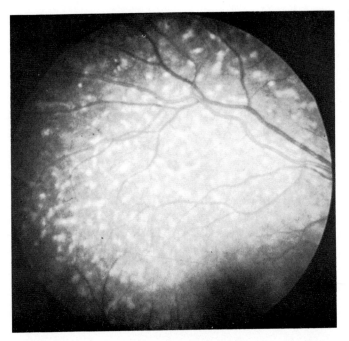

FIG. 3-16. Fundus flavimaculatus in a young woman. The lesions have pisciform appearance, in contrast to the more globular appearance of drusen. Usually these lesions end at or just before the equator.

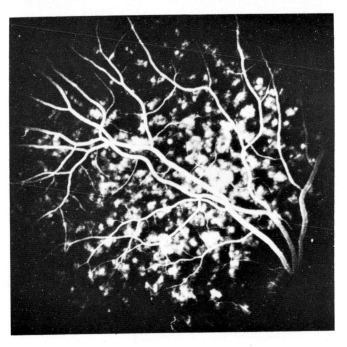

FIG. 3-17. Fluorescein angiography of the patient in Figure 3-16 shows that some areas transmit fluorescein while others obscure the transmission of the dye.

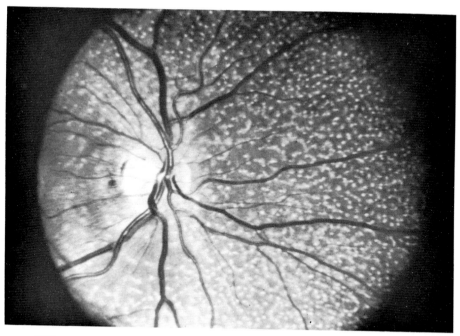

FIG. 3-18. Fundus albipunctata, showing the small white dots throughout the fundus in the posterior pole.

FIG. 3-19. The dots of fundus albipunctata extending into the periphery. This is a nonprogressive disease, in contrast to retinitis punctata albescens, which leads to night blindness.

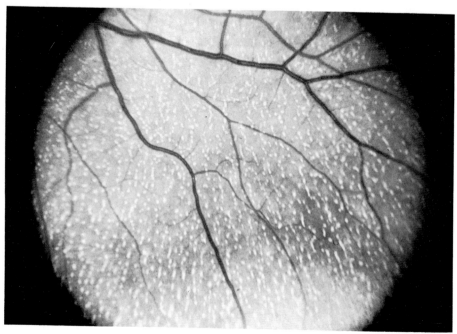

GYRATE ATROPHY

Gyrate atrophy, a slow, progressive, patchy atrophy of the choroid, pigment epithelium, and retina, starts in the periphery but eventually involves all of the fundus (Figs. 3-20, 3-21, and 3-22). Night blindness and gradually increasing visual failure are prominent symptoms.

Gyrate atrophy has been confused with choroideremia because of the similar appearance of the fundus in the final stages. However, there is a clear difference in the mode of inheritance, since gyrate atrophy is carried as a recessive trait. Usually there is no problem in differentiating gyrate atrophy from progressive myopia because myopic changes tend to be concentrated at the posterior pole, whereas those in gyrate atrophy originate in the periphery. Furthermore, night blindness and significant visual field abnormalities are less common in progressive myopia.

Recently the enzymatic aberration hyperornithinemia has been associated with cases of gyrate atrophy, and investigation into special diets is underway to see whether or not diet can influence the course of the disease.[14, 15] The basic metabolic defect is a deficiency of the enzyme ornithine transcarbamylase, which results in hyperornithemia.

VARIED MODES OF INHERITANCE

RETINITIS PIGMENTOSA

Retinitis pigmentosa, or primary pigmentary dystrophy of the retina, is a condition that deserves separate consideration because of its pleomorphic nature and the fact that it may be inherited as either an X-linked recessive, autosomal dominant, or autosomal recessive condition. Of these, the X-linked variety is probably the most disabling, and the recessive the most common. Sporadic cases may also occur. Named retinitis pigmentosa by Donders[5] in 1855, the condition is probably more accurately called pigmentary retinal dystrophy.

Fundus Characteristics

Retinitis pigmentosa is characterized by progressive deterioration of night vision and peripheral field. Clinically, a narrowing of the retinal vessels, waxy pallor of the optic disc, and the appearance, initially at the equator, of "bone spicule" ("bone corpuscle") pigment (Fig. 3-23) constitute typical findings. Late in the disease, atrophy of the retinal pigment epithelium may also occur. The condition is always bilateral in hereditary cases. Unilateral occurrences do not represent true retinitis pigmentosa, but are more likely explained by retinal vascular problems. Pigmentary changes typically become visible during the first decade of life, beginning as fine dots which gradually assume a spidery bone corpuscle appearance. As the disease progresses, the equatorial girdle widens and a ring scotoma is produced in the

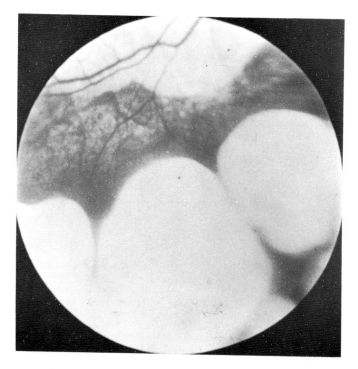

FIG. 3-20. Gyrate atrophy, usually inherited as an autosomal recessive condition, begins in the fundus periphery.

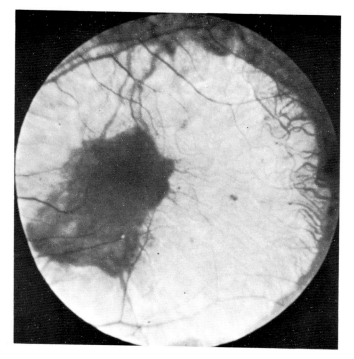

FIG. 3-21. Later gyrate atrophy can extend into the posterior pole.

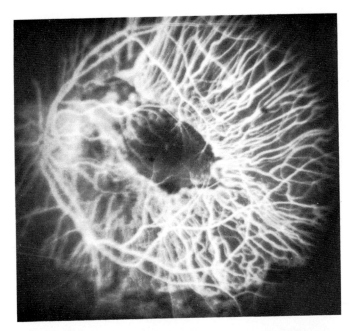

FIG. 3-22. Fluorescein angiography in gyrate atrophy shows absence of pigment epithelium and choriocapillaris with only preservation of the large choroidal vessels.

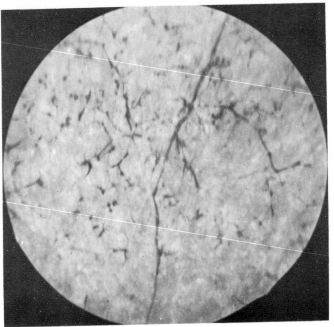

FIG. 3-23. Typical appearance of the "bone spicule" pigmentary changes in retinitis pigmentosa.

visual field. Atypical pigmentary variations may occur in which pigment is sparse or absent, as in retinitis pigmentosa sine pigmento.[10]

Electroretinographic Changes

The ERG is of great importance in the diagnosis. In primary pigmentary degeneration of the retina, the ERG response is subnormal or absent, a change which appears before the subjective visual deterioration or the ophthalmoscopically visible changes.

Histologic Findings

Histologic study reveals a general disappearance of the neuroepithelial elements, proliferation of glial cells, changes in the pigment epithelium, and an obliterative sclerosis of the retinal vessels.[1, 6] First to be affected are the rods, in contrast to the ganglion cells and the nerve fiber layer, which may remain unaffected even when the eye is blind. The migration of pigment into the retina, aided by macrophages, follows the degeneration.[10]

Electron microscopic studies suggest that the first changes entail destruction of the basement membrane and the básal infoldings of the pigment epithelium. Cone remnants appear as "finger-ring" lamellar masses and may be fragmented. Cells of the pigment epithelium show narrowing and their nuclei come to rest close to the basement membrane. Mitochondria are sparse in these cells.

Differential Diagnosis

Laurence-Moon-Biedl Syndrome. Many conditions are associated with retinitis pigmentosa–like fundus changes (Table 3-2). Perhaps one of the best known is the Laurence-Moon-Biedl syndrome[13] (also known as Laurence-Moon-Bardet-Biedl syndrome), which embraces the combination of mental retardation, hypogenitalism, obesity, polydactyly (Fig. 3-24), and, frequently, retinal changes. The syndrome shows a recessive inheritance pattern,[13] and males predominate. The retinal changes may simulate typical retinitis pigmentosa or may be characterized by macular degeneration. A third form appears as a disseminated choroidal sclerosis. About 85 percent of the patients with Laurence-Moon-Biedl syndrome will show abnormalities of the ERG, but only 15 percent will have the typical pigmentary changes of the retina seen in retinitis pigmentosa.

Refsum's Disease and Abetalipoproteinemia (Bassen-Kornzweig Syndrome). The two autosomal recessive conditions, Refsum's disease—i.e., polyneuritis, atypical pigmentary degeneration, cardiac anomalies, cerebellar ataxia, and paresis of the lower extremities—and abetalipoproteinemia (Bassen-Kornzweig syndrome)—i.e., spinocerebellar degeneration, low blood cholesterol, celiac disease, and betalipoprotein deficiency—should also be mentioned in the differential diagnosis since the ERG is diminished or

TABLE 3-2
Some Hereditary Conditions Associated with Retinitis Pigmentosa

Disorder	Inheritance Pattern	Other Findings
Laurence-Moon-Biedl Syndrome	Autosomal recessive	Mental retardation, polydactyly, obesity, hypogenitalism, deafness
Refsum's Disease	Autosomal recessive	Polyneuropathy, ataxia, increased phytanic acid, deafness
Cockayne's Syndrome	Autosomal recessive	Dwarfism, precocious senility, mental retardation, deafness
Goldmann-Favré	Autosomal recessive	Cataracts, optically empty vitreous cavity
Hallgren's	Autosomal recessive	Retinoschisis, retinal detachment, cerebellar ataxia
Usher's Syndrome	Autosomal recessive	Deafness
Bassen-Kornzweig Syndrome	Autosomal recessive	Acanthocytosis, abetalipoproteinemia, ataxia
Friedreich's Ataxia	Autosomal recessive	Posterior column disease, nystagmus, ataxia
Pelizaeus-Merzbacher Disease	X-Linked recessive	Spasticity, cerebellar ataxia, dementia, "wandering eyes"
Mucopolysaccharidosis Type I (Hurler's Syndrome)	Autosomal recessive	Gargoylism, corneal clouding, mental retardation
Type II (Hunter's Syndrome)	X-Linked recessive	Mental retardation, skeletal abnormalities, hepatosplenogemaly
Type III (Sanfilippo's Syndrome)	Autosomal recessive	Mental retardation
Type IV (Morquio's Syndrome)	Autosomal recessive	Skeletal abnormalities, corneal clouding

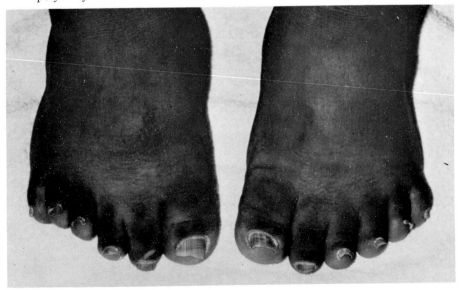

FIG. 3-24. A young man with Laurence-Moon-Biedl syndrome showing polydactylism.

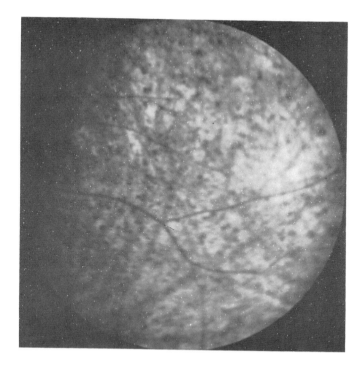

FIG. 3-25. Rubella retinopathy (pseudoretinitis pigmentosa). Note the typical salt-and-pepper appearance due to changes in the pigment epithelium.

absent in these conditions and pigmentary retinal changes occur. In addition, patients with abetalipoproteinemia have changes in their erythrocytes, characterized by crenation and spiny projections (acanthocytosis). This is the one disease associated with retinitis pigmentosa that is treatable: some of these patients benefit from high doses of vitamin A.

Hallgren's and Cockayne's Syndromes. Hallgren's syndrome and Cockayne's syndrome are also autosomal recessive disorders, both of which are associated with retinitis pigmentosa, and with deafness and mental deficiency. Cerebellar ataxia is common to Hallgren's syndrome, while Cockayne's syndrome is characterized by a progerialike dwarfism.

Rubella Retinopathy. The retinopathy resulting from congenital rubella may also cause some confusion in the differential diagnosis of retinitis pigmentosa. The fundus in rubella retinopathy typically presents a widespread mottled or blotchy appearance, with hyperpigmented or normally pigmented areas alternating with depigmented areas that show considerable variation in size. This type of picture is often referred to as a salt-and-pepper pigmentation of the fundus, or pseudoretinitis pigmentosa (Fig. 3-25; see also Figs. 5-17 and 5-18 in Chap. 5). The pigment alteration usually is most marked in the posterior pole, and especially in the macula, where the pigment clumping tends to be much coarser than the dustlike pigmentation seen in the periphery. Rarely, the peripheral retina may be more involved than the posterior portion. Rubella retinopathy in no way resembles the acute infiltrative lesions that accompany other viral infections such as herpes simplex, Behcet's syndrome, or cytomegalic inclusion disease. Segmental distribution and unilateral involvement may also be seen. The retinal vessels are not

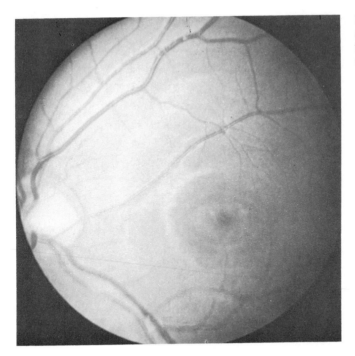

FIG. 3-26. Typical appearance of a bull's-eye the macula secondary to chloroquine retinopathy.

involved and appear normal, as does the ERG. Generally the eye is not adversely affected physiologically.

Although the retinopathy of rubella syndrome tends to remain stationary under normal circumstances, this static state may be dramatically changed following intraocular surgery. Following cataract or iridic surgery, a series of events may occasionally occur which ultimately lead to total retinal detachment and phthisis bulbi. In these eyes there first seems to be a marked postoperative nongranulomatous, inflammatory reaction in the area of the lens remnants, the iris, or both. The ciliary body then becomes involved in the reaction. A cyclitic membrane forms and ultimately, with contracture of this membrane, retinal detachment results. Persistent rubella virus, liberated by the surgery, is apparently responsible for setting off the above series of events. The reparative process of the eye, mainly the formation of granulation tissue, leads to the devastating intraocular complications of cyclitic membrane and retinal detachment.[20]

Syphilis. In syphilis a salt-and-pepper fundus may also occur which closely resembles that seen in rubella. The resemblance is most marked when the pigment deposits in the syphilitic retina are fine and diffusely scattered; usually, however, they are more marked peripherally although sometimes they may best be seen posteriorly. These changes are typically seen in congenital syphilis but may be observed in the acquired disease as well. The ERG is very helpful in differentiating between retinitis pigmentosa and syphilis. When retinitis pigmentosa is associated with pigment changes as severe as in syphilis, the ERG is flat. In syphilis it is reduced but present.

Drug Toxicities. Phenothiazines and chloroquine therapy can also lead to retinal pigmentary disturbances. In both instances the change is dose- and time-related. For example, the typical macular bull's-eye appearance in chloroquine retinopathy is uncommon with a total dosage of less than 100 grams. However, with administration of 300 grams of chloroquine the risks of retinopathy increase significantly (Fig. 3-26). Cessation of the medication once the retinopathy has developed does not lead to its disappearance—it may even progress.

Cystinosis. In 1967 Wong, Lietman, and Seegmiller[19] described retinal changes in juvenile cystinosis (Lignac-Fanconi syndrome) that were not seen in adults. The presence of corneal crystals is well known in this condition. Fundus changes consist of generalized depigmentation in the retinal periphery associated with adjacent pigment clumping varying in size from 1/10 of a disc diameter to fine pepperlike stippling. The patients ranged in age from 5 weeks to 7 years and all demonstrated changes in the pigment epithelium. The lesions were usually symmetrical in both eyes and involved the entire retinal periphery. Clinically, the fundus changes consisted of a generalized depigmentation which was often patchy. Superimposed on this light background were pigment clumps which varied in size from about 1/10 disc diameter to a very fine pepperlike stippling. Occasionally, the pigment formed small ringlets. The intensity of the pigmentation tended to fade posteriorly so that the region behind the equator was generally devoid of abnormal pigmentation.

REFERENCES

1. **Alezzandrine A:** Retinitis pigmentosa en Sectores Simmetricos, Archivos De Oftalmologia. 40:72–75, 1965
2. **Berson EL:** Electroretinographic testing as an aid in determining visual progress in families with hereditary retinal degeneration. In Allen HF (ed): Retina Congress. New York, Appleton-Century-Crofts, 1972, pp 41–54
3. **Cohen AM:** Lessons from diabetes in Yemenites. Isr J Med Sci 7:1554–1557, 1971
4. **Cross HE:** The nosology of hereditary retinal diseases. Ophthalmol Dig 39:13–21, 1977
5. **Donders FC:** Betriage zur pathogisher anatomie des auges. Albrecht von Graefes Arch Klin Ophthalmol 1:106–118, 1855
6. **Duke-Elder S:** Diseases of the Retina, Vol X. St. Louis, Mosby 1967
7. **Franceschetti A:** A special form of tapeoretinal degeneration: fundus flavimaculatus. Trans Am Acad Ophthalmol Otolaryngol 69:1048–1053, 1965
8. **Freeman H:** In Tasman W (ed): Retinal Diseases in Children. New York, Harper & Row, 1971, pp 1–18
9. **Gass JDM:** Steroscopic Atlas of Macular Diseases. St. Louis, Mosby, 1970, p 124
10. **Hogan MJ, Zimmerman LT:** Ophthalmic Pathology, 2nd ed. Philadelphia, Saunders, 1962, p 543
11. **Jansen L:** Degeneratio hyaloideo-retinalis hereditaria. Ophthalmologica 144:458, 1962
12. **Kimura SJ, Caygill WM (eds):** Retinal Disease. Symposium on differential diagnostic problems of posterior uveitis. Philadelphia, Lea & Febiger, 1969, p 131
12a. **Klien BA, Krill AE:** Fundus flavimaculatus. Clinical, functional, and histopathologic observations. Am J Ophthalmol 64:3–23, 1967
13. **Lawrence JL, Moon RD:** Four cases of retinitis pigmentosa occurring in the same family and accompanied by general imperfections in development. Ophthalmol Rev 2:32–41, 1866
13a. **Lucier A, Eagle R:** Personal communication.
14. **McCulloch C, Marliss E:** Gyrate atrophy of the choroid and retina: clinical, ophthalmologic, and biochemical considerations. Trans Am Ophthalmol Soc 73:163–171, 1975

15. **McCulloch JC, Arshinoff S, Marliss E, and Parker J:** Hyperornithinemia and gyrate atrophy of choroid and retina. Trans Am Ophthalmol Soc 85:918–928, 1978

15a. **O'Donnell FE Jr, King RA, Green WR, et al.:** Autosomal recessively inherited ocular albinism. Arch Ophthalmol 96:1621–1625, 1978

15b. **Opitz JM:** Ocular abnormalities in malformation syndromes. Trans Amer Acad Ophthal and Otol, 76:1193–1202, 1972.

16. **Stargardt K:** Ueber familiare, progressive degeneration in der Makulagegend des Auges. Albrecht von Graefes Arch Klin Ophthalmol 7:534, 1909

17. **Stickler GB, Belau PG, Farrell FJ, Jones JD, Pugh DG, Steinberg AG, Ward LE:** Hereditary progressive arthro-ophthalmopathy. Mayo Clin Proc 40:433–455, 1965

18. **Wagner H:** Ein Bisher unbekanntes Erbleiden des Auges (Degeneratio hyaloideroretinalis hereditoria) beobachtet im Kanton Zurich. Klin Monatsbl Augenheilkd 100:840–856, 1938

19. **Wong VG, Lietman PS, Seegmiller JE:** Alterations of pigment epithelium in cystenosis. Arch Ophthalmol 77:361–370, 1967

20. **Yanoff M:** The retina in rubella. In Tasman W (ed): Retinal Diseases in Children. New York, Harper & Row, 1971, pp 223–232

21. **Yanoff M, Rahn KK, Zimmerman LE:** Histopathy of juvenile retinoschisis. Arch Ophthalmol 79:49–53, 1968

4

Developmental
Abnormalities

It is somewhat unusual for developmental abnormalities of the eye to involve the peripheral fundus exclusively. Certain developmental conditions, however, may be more common or more pronounced in the peripheral retina or choroid. This chapter considers some of the more clinically important nonhereditary developmental abnormalities affecting the peripheral fundus. Congenital conditions with a hereditary basis are discussed in Chapter 3. Other developmental conditions which have little clinical significance and which are considered merely anatomical variations are discussed in Chapter 1.

PERSISTENT HYPERPLASTIC PRIMARY VITREOUS

Persistent hyperplastic primary vitreous (PHPV) is an abnormal persistence and proliferation of the primary vitreous.[16] It occurs unilaterally in a microphthalmic eye. In contrast to retrolental fibroplasia (retinopathy of prematurity, RLF; see in Chap. 6), it is usually detected at birth in a full-term baby.[12] Although the etiology and pathogenesis are poorly understood, the clinical and pathologic features were well described by Reese.[13] Two rather distinct forms of PHPV are recognized and are designated as the anterior and the posterior types.

ANTERIOR TYPE

Clinical Features and Variations

Anterior PHPV may encompass a wide spectrum of clinical findings ranging from mild to very severe. The mild form may be represented as a dense white

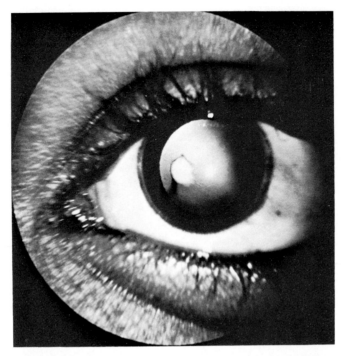

FIG. 4-1. Mild anterior persistent hyperplastic primary vitreous (PHPV) showing an opacity on t posterior surface of the **l**

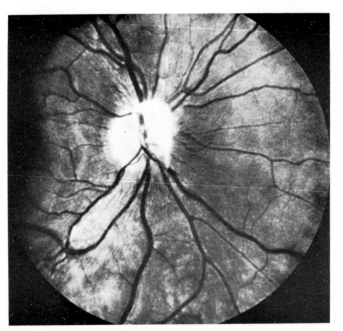

FIG. 4-2. Fundus photograph of a Bergmeister's papilla, representing a mild form persistence of the poster hyaloid system.

opacity on the posterior surface of the lens, somewhat larger than a Mittendorf's dot (Fig. 4-1). Such mild cases may show either a persistent hyaloid artery or a Bergmeister's papilla on the optic disc (Fig. 4-2).

The moderately severe form is characterized by a dense white opacity in the retrolental area. It is often attached to the posterior lens capsule. In contrast to the findings in the mild form, ophthalmoscopy may reveal peripapillary retinal detachment or pigmentary changes. There is frequently a hyaloid artery, with connective tissue extending from the optic disc to the retrolental mass (Fig. 4-3). Clinically, the involved eye may appear microphthalmic, a finding which may be confirmed with ultrasonography.

The severe form of PHPV is characterized by a yellowish white retrolental mass which is often obscured by a dense cataract, precluding any view of the fundus (Fig. 4-4). There is usually rather severe microphthalmia with a shallow anterior chamber. Prominent, often vascularized, pupillary membranes may extend from the iris collarette across the anterior surface of the lens (Fig. 4-5).When the pupil is widely dilated, the ciliary processes may be easily visualized at the lens equator. This results from traction of the retrolental mass, which causes the ciliary processes to be displaced centrally. Other associated clinical findings, including corectopia, subluxated lens, and uveal or optic colobomas, have also been recognized.[7]

Clinical Course

The clinical course of anterior PHPV may also, like the severity, be variable. The mild form is often nonprogressive and may remain stationary for many months. The more advanced forms, however, may produce a number of complications. One of the earliest complications is cataract formation. This occurs secondary to a dehiscence in the posterior lens capsule, leading to progressive opacification. Blood vessels from the retrolental tissue may invade the lens. In some cases the cataract may undergo spontaneous resolution, with clearing of the central portion, leaving only folded capsular remnants.

Another complication is secondary narrow-angle glaucoma. As the retrolental mass and cataract become larger, the anterior chamber becomes more shallow, causing a compromise of the aqueous outflow. If the glaucoma occurs early in infancy the globe may enlarge, converting the eye from microphthalmic to normal size or even to buphthalmic.

A third complication is retinal detachment. The retrolental mass may exert considerable traction on the fundus periphery, leading to either a nonrhegmatogenous or a rhegmatogenous retinal detachment (see Chap. 9), which may eventually become total (Fig. 4-6). In such cases successful treatment is often impossible.

Pathology

The histopathology of PHPV is sometimes difficult to interpret because the globe is often distorted from the numerous complications by the time it is

(Text continues on page 66)

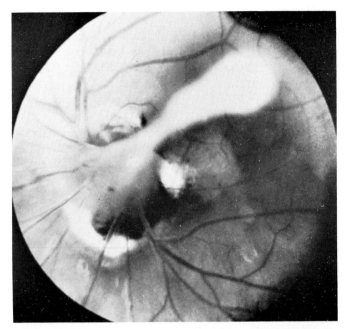

FIG. 4-3. Moderately seve form of anterior PHPV wi hyaloid remnants over the disc and with peripapilla pigment proliferation.

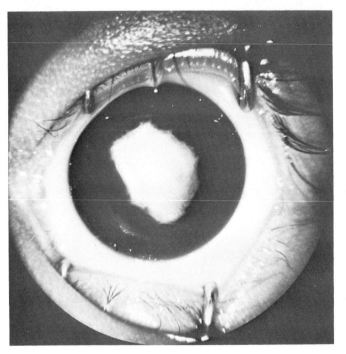

FIG. 4-4. Severe form of PHPV showing a dense w retrolental mass.

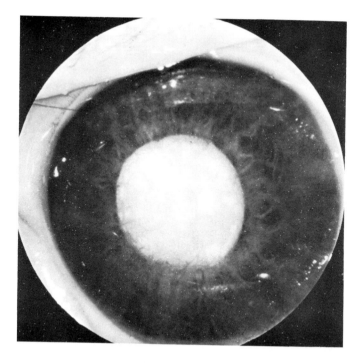

FIG. 4-5. Vascularized pupillary membranes in PHPV.

FIG. 4-6. Sectioned eye with PHPV. Note the dense retrolental mass and the total retinal detachment. (AFIP accession no. 1387755)

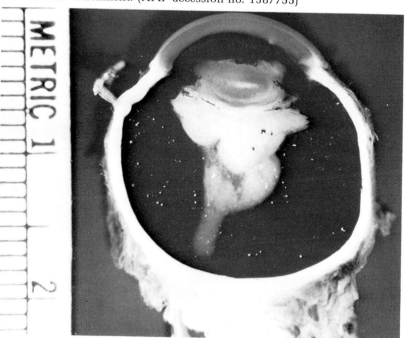

enucleated. In some cases which have been enucleated as suspected retinoblastoma, the histologic features are more clearly defined.

The eye is usually smaller than normal in anteroposterior diameter. Sectioning reveals a white retrolental mass, often associated with a shallow anterior chamber and a cataract. A persistent hyaloid artery is common, often associated with dense connective tissue, and extending from the retrolental mass to the optic disc (Fig. 4-7). The ciliary processes, and sometimes the peripheral retina, are often pulled into the retrolental mass.

Microscopic examination reveals characteristic findings in cases of PHPV (Fig. 4-8). There is loose fibrovascular tissue in the retrolental area, which may contain cartilage, fat, or glial tissue.[12] The peripheral portion of the mass may contain ciliary epithelium and sensory retina as a result of traction (Fig. 4-8). The lens may be shrunken and calcified, sometimes with intralenticular lipid which can be demonstrated with special stains. Preretinal glial nodules, thought to represent neuroectodermal proliferation, have also been observed histologically in PHPV.[1, 7] Dysplastic retina, characterized by tubular rosettes, may also be present.

Pathogenesis

The pathogenesis of PHPV is poorly understood. In most cases the birth history is normal, with no known previous infection or trauma. One may speculate that some type of ocular insult occurs during embryologic development which prevents both resolution of the primary vitreous and development of the secondary vitreous. Manschot described the presence of preretinal glial tissue in nine of ten cases of PHPV studied histologically.[7] He found identical structures in a presumably normal 35-mm. embryo. Since the secondary vitreous is a neuroectodermal structure originating from Muller's cells, perhaps the insult occurs at about the 35-mm. stage, when the secondary vitreous should be developing from the footplates of Muller's cells. This could result in an arrest in the development of the secondary vitreous, with persistence of the primary vitreous. Why the persistent primary vitreous undergoes proliferation in some cases is still unclear.

Differential Diagnosis

The differential diagnosis of anterior PHPV includes any of the causes of a white pupillary reflex in a child, a subject which is covered in Chapter 7 under Retinoblastoma.

The most important lesion to differentiate from anterior PHPV is retinoblastoma. In contrast to retinoblastoma, PHPV is present at birth and almost always occurs unilaterally in a microphthalmic eye. It is usually associated with a cataract, while the lens is usually clear in eyes with retinoblastoma. PHPV is associated with severe tractional phenomena, as suggested by the elongated ciliary processes and tractional retinal detachment. Evidence of vitreous traction is rare with retinoblastoma.

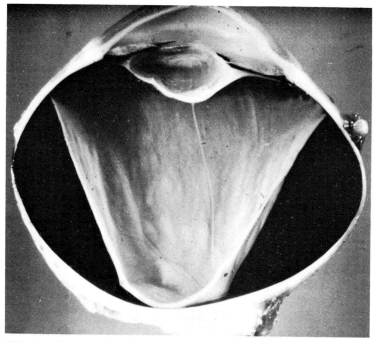

FIG. 4-7. Sectioned globe with PHPV showing a retrolental mass and persistent hyaloid artery. (AFIP accession no. 786570)

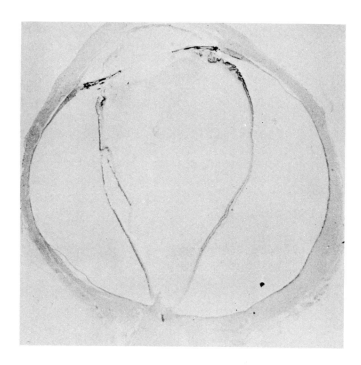

FIG. 4-8. Histologic section of a globe with PHPV. The eye was microphthalmic. (AFIP accession no. 974652)

Treatment

A number of years ago, PHPV was untreatable in most cases. With improvements in vitreous surgery some cases can now be successfully treated, although good visual results are the exception rather than the rule.

The mild form of PHPV, characterized by a small posterior lens opacity, hyaloid artery, and normal fundus, probably should not be treated surgically. The use of mydriatics may keep the pupil dilated, allowing the child to have some vision around the opacity. Less commonly, an optical iridectomy may be tried. If the child has reasonably good vision in the involved eye, occlusion of the opposite eye to minimize amblyopia may be considered.

In more advanced cases in which progressive traction is present, or in cases where ultrasonography has demonstrated an early retinal detachment, excision of the retrolental mass may be necessary. This usually involves removal of the lens, thus rendering the child aphakic.

Some of the early surgical attempts to remove PHPV involved a limbal incision with a direct approach to remove the fibrovascular mass.[4] An anterior vitrectomy was performed, using cellulose sponges and fine scissors. With the advent of closed intraocular microsurgery, surgeons began to use various closed methods with either a pars plana or a limbal approach. In many cases the cataractous lens is so dense and membranous that a limbal incision with linear extraction is necessary. No large series has been reported, but because the involved eye often has microphthalmia and other abnormalities, excellent visual results should not be expected in all cases. The goal of treatment should be to relieve the vitreous traction and to stabilize the eye in hopes of preventing retinal detachment, glaucoma, phthisis, and other complications.

POSTERIOR TYPE

The posterior type of PHPV differs from the anterior type in its clinical features, clinical course, and differential diagnosis.[10] Although this condition, sometimes called falciform fold or congenital retinal fold, has been attributed to persistence of the primary vitreous, this remains somewhat controversial. It is now widely recognized that certain specific conditions, such as RLF or nematode granuloma, may produce a similar clinical picture (see Differential Diagnosis, below).

Clinical Features and Variations

As with the anterior type, the clinical features of posterior PHPV also form a spectrum ranging from mild to severe. The condition is unilateral in 83 percent of cases and bilateral in 17 percent.[9] The anterior segment is not markedly abnormal, although about half of the patients have some degree of microcornea, and lens opacities are occasionally present.

Most of the significant pathologic changes are confined to the posterior pole. The mild form may demonstrate only excessive mesodermal elements over the optic disc and a small peripapillary retinal detachment. The more advanced form, however, is associated with severe vitreoretinal traction, which forms a vascularized fibroglial fold that passes from the optic disc towards the peripheral fundus (Fig. 4-9A). In many cases there is dense white tissue at the vitreoretinal interface, corresponding to the anterior extent of the fold (Fig. 4-9B).

Clinical Course

The mild form of posterior PHPV may remain stationary for many years with no signs of progression. The more advanced type, associated with a large retinal fold, may lead to a localized or extensive retinal detachment which may be difficult to repair with conventional surgery.

Pathology

Few cases of posterior PHPV have been examined histologically. The fold is reported to contain persistent hyaloid vessels and dysplastic retinal rosettes.[6, 10] The sensory retina may show extensive degenerative changes, but the retinal pigment epithelium is usually normal.

Differential Diagnosis

The differential diagnosis of posterior PHPV includes retinoblastoma, RLF, familial exudative vitreoretinopathy, nematode granuloma, and trauma either with or without an intraocular foreign body.

Retinoblastoma (see in Chap. 7), as previously mentioned, is not associated with extensive vitreoretinal traction, and its other well-known features should present little diagnostic difficulty. In RLF (see in Chap. 6), the history of prematurity and of oxygen therapy, combined with bilateral findings, should be helpful in the differentiation. It is important, however, to note that RLF may occasionally be unilateral in patients who received no oxygen. In familial exudative vitreoretinopathy (see differential diagnosis of Coats' disease, in Chap. 6), the findings are bilateral, the family history is often positive, and there may be more exudation.

Nematode granuloma (see Nematode Endophthalmitis in Chap. 5) may produce a unilateral retinal fold, making it difficult to differentiate from posterior PHPV. The history of contact with puppies and the typical laboratory findings may be helpful, although in some cases the diagnosis remains in doubt. In cases of trauma or intraocular foreign body, a history of injury associated with radiologic or ultrasonographic evidence of a foreign body should be helpful.

Treatment

In contrast to anterior PHPV, there is no specific treatment for posterior PHPV. If the retinal detachment should progress, then conventional retinal detachment surgery may be utilized. If vitreous traction bands are present, closed

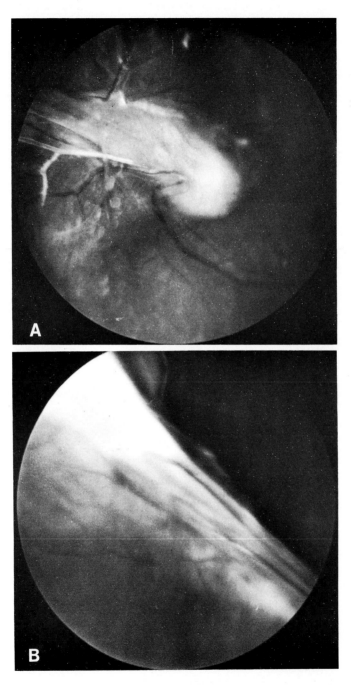

FIG. 4-9. Posterior PHPV. A fibrovascular mass exten from the disc towards the nasal periphery. **B.** Nasal periphery of the same eye showing termination of th fibrovascular tissue at the serrata.

intraocular microsurgery may be attempted, to release the vitreous traction on the retina, but the chances of visual improvement are minimal.

COLOBOMA

The coloboma is a rather common developmental abnormality. It is bilateral in about half the cases. Although an isolated lesion in the macular area may occur, the majority involve the iris and the peripheral fundus. The coloboma may occur as a rather common, typical type which is located in the inferonasal quadrant or as a rare, atypical type which may be located in any other quadrant.

Clinical Features

The patient's central vision may range from normal to markedly diminished, depending on the location and the extent of the lesion. The typical inferior or inferonasal coloboma appears as a depressed yellowish white area which is well delineated and often has a clumping of pigment on the margin. It usually extends from the ciliary body region for a variable distance posteriorly. The more advanced coloboma may incorporate the optic disc and the macular area. Choroidal or retinal blood vessels are frequently present within the involved area (Fig. 4-10). The lesion is often associated with an iris or lens coloboma in the same quadrant (Fig. 4-11). The lens coloboma is probably due to an absence of zonules in the area of the coloboma, which leads to a lack of zonular support for the lens in the involved quadrant.

Pathology

The pathology of the coloboma is variable, but is usually characterized by an absence or marked thinning of both the sensory retina and the choroid. The nuclear layers and pigment epithelium usually come to a rather abrupt end at the margin. The retinal pigment epithelium is often folded and thickened, explaining the hyperpigmentation seen ophthalmoscopically. The central portion of the coloboma may show only sclera covered by thin connective tissue which appears continuous with the nerve fiber layer. The residual retina may be dysplastic (see Retinal Dysplasia, below). A few retinal blood vessels may be present within this tissue (Fig. 4-12).

The sclera may be of normal thickness, but it is often thinned in the area of the coloboma, allowing the intraocular contents to bulge outward. This can lead to either a staphylomatous lesion or an orbital cyst in the involved quadrant.

Pathogenesis

During the embryonic development of the eye there is a cleft or fissure, located inferonasally, which allows the hyaloid vessels to enter the eye. During

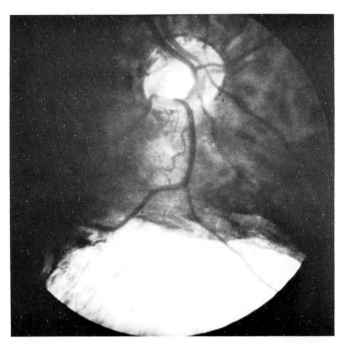

FIG. 4-10. Coloboma of the choroid inferior to the optic disc.

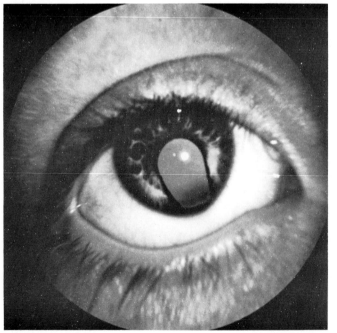

FIG. 4-11. Coloboma of the iris. Note the inferonasal location.

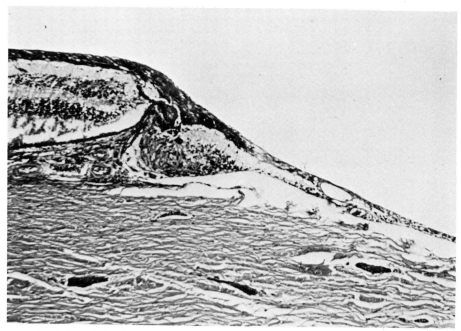

FIG. 4-12. Histologic section of a choroidal coloboma. Note the thin retinal and choroidal remnants over the sclera on the right. (Wilmer Eye Institute Pathology no. 31921; Courtesy of Dr. W. R. Green) (Hematoxylin-eosin stain; × 75)

normal development, this fissure becomes closed by fusion of the two layers of the optic cup. The process of fusion begins in the equatorial area and proceeds anteriorly and posteriorly. When fusion is complete, the retina and choroid appear normal. If fusion is incomplete, defects in these tissues occur and lead to a typical coloboma.[3]

While the mechanism for the development of a typical coloboma is thus understood, its cause is not clear. The association of coloboma with chromosomal defects such as trisomy 13 and trisomy 18, as well as with toxic conditions such as thalidomide toxicity, suggest that a variety of diversified ocular insults may lead to this condition.

The atypical coloboma, which may occur in any quadrant, is very rare and its mechanism of development is poorly understood. In some cases an isolated macular coloboma may occur. Its mechanism is also unclear, but some of these cases may represent inactive congenital toxoplasmosis.

Differential Diagnosis

The diagnosis of coloboma should be relatively easy in most cases because of its classic appearance. Larger lesions may produce a white pupillary reflex, or leukocoria, and retinoblastoma must therefore be excluded. The use of indirect ophthalmoscopy will demonstrate the depressed rather than elevated configuration.

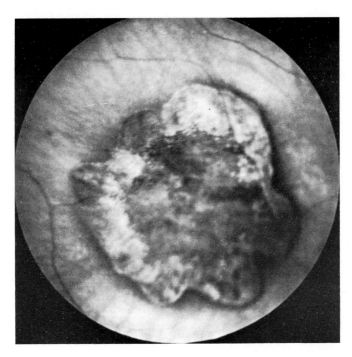

FIG. 4-13. Fundus photograph of the solitary type of congenital hypertrophy of the retinal pigment epithelium. Although the lesion is flat it gives the impression of being elevated.

Inflammatory lesions such as toxoplasmic chorioretinitis (see Toxoplasmosis in Chap. 5) should also be considered in the differential diagnosis. However, most inflammatory scars are smaller and are multifocal. As previously mentioned, some cases of macular coloboma may represent inactive macular toxoplasmosis.

Treatment

No treatment is available for coloboma. The condition is usually nonprogressive, although complications such as retinal detachment may occur. If a detachment does occur, the retinal break may lie within the colobomatous area and may therefore be very difficult to visualize.[5] A conventional scleral buckling procedure should be used to treat the detachment, but the visual prognosis is much worse than for routine rhegmatogenous detachments.

HYPERTROPHY OF THE RETINAL PIGMENT EPITHELIUM

In some eyes, one or more dark plaques may be found anywhere in the fundus at the level of the retinal pigment epithelium. This condition has been called congenital hypertrophy of the retinal pigment epithelium (CHRPE). It may occur as a solitary lesion or it may be multifocal, an entity called congenital grouped pigmentation, or "bear tracks." It is now widely recognized that these two conditions are the same histologically and should therefore be classified together.

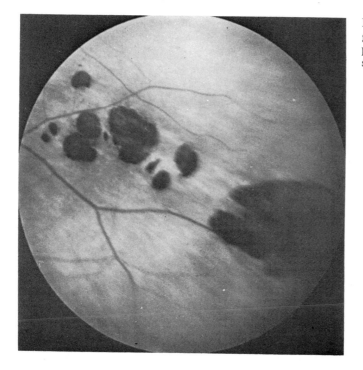

FIG. 4-14. Congenital grouped pigmentation in the peripheral fundus. Note the similarity to animal tracks.

SOLITARY TYPE

Clinical Features

The solitary type of CHRPE (Fig. 4-13) is usually asymptomatic and is discovered on routine ocular examination.[11] It appears ophthalmoscopically as a flat, well-delineated lesion which is usually a dark black, although it may contain areas of depigmentation. These areas may be so extensive that the entire lesion may appear amelanotic. The lesion is usually 1 or 2 disc diameters in size when found in the posterior pole, but is often much larger when found in the periphery. The peripheral lesions sometimes give the false impression of being elevated when examined with indirect ophthalmoscopy.

The areas of depigmentation on the lesion may resemble drusen. There is sometimes a depigmented halo surrounding the mass. Fluorescein angiography shows early hypofluorescence of the pigmented portions of the lesion and relative hyperfluorescence of the depigmented areas. There is no late staining with the dye. Usually, CHRPE is a stationary lesion with no tendency to grow. In rare instances, however, the lesion has been observed to enlarge slowly over a long period of time.[8]

Pathology

Pathologically, CHRPE is characterized by a local area of hyperpigmentation within an otherwise normal RPE. Although the hyperpigmented RPE cells are only one layer in thickness, they are often taller than normal and contain more pigment granules. The granules are usually larger and more globular than in the normal RPE adjacent to the lesion. The islands of depigmentation represent focal areas in which a group of RPE cells are lacking in pigment granules. The surrounding halo shows a similar lack of pigmentation histologically. The overlying sensory retina may sometimes exhibit degenerative changes which account for the scotomas that are occasionally detectable.[2]

Differential Diagnosis

The differential diagnosis of solitary CHRPE includes choroidal melanoma and choroidal nevus (see in Chap. 7), reactive hyperplasia of the RPE (see in Chap. 7), hemorrhagic detachment of the RPE, and the black sunburst sign of sickle cell retinopathy (see Fig. 6-8 in Chap. 8). The specific differential features are discussed in the literature.[11] The flat, well-delineated appearance of this condition, and the depigmented foci and halo, should easily differentiate it from the other conditions.

MULTIFOCAL TYPE

Congenital grouped pigmentation appears as a variable number of groups of pigmented plaques, often involving a sector of the fundus. The area of involvement becomes wider toward the periphery. Each group may have a larger lesion surrounded by several smaller ones, resembling the paws and toes of an animal footprint; hence the term "bear-track" pigmentation (Fig. 4-14).

Both the solitary and multifocal types of CHRPE demonstrate the same histologic features. They therefore appear to represent different clinical expressions of the same pathologic entity.

The differential diagnosis of multifocal CHRPE includes sector retinitis pigmentosa (see in Chap. 3) and any cause of pigment dispersion, such as trauma or inflammation. Its appearance is usually quite typical and the diagnosis is not difficult.

RETINAL DYSPLASIA

This condition is included here for completeness, although retinal dysplasia is not a specific disease entity. It is, rather, a term which describes certain histopathologic findings that may occur in a number of clinical situations.

Pathology

Retinal dysplasia is characterized by areas of malformed retina with loss of the regular architecture. The most characteristic feature is the well-differentiated tubular or branching retinal rosette, quite different from the uniform round

Flexner-Wintersteiner rosette of retinoblastoma[15] (see Fig. 7-7, in Chap. 7). It is noteworthy that the dysplasia is most severe in areas where the developing sensory retina has been separated from the retinal pigment epithelium for any of several reasons.[18]

Associated Entities

Eyes with histologic features of retinal dysplasia have been seen in association with a diversity of clinical entities. The most widely recognized is trisomy 13, sometimes called Patau's syndrome or the Reese-Blodi-Straatsma syndrome.[14, 15] Although the clinical manifestations may vary, the patient usually has bilaterally malformed retinas with dysplasia, coloboma, cataracts, and other changes. This syndrome is often fatal as a result of the numerous associated systemic and central nervous system malformations. Retinal dysplasia has also been observed in conjunction with PHPV of both the anterior and posterior types, as well as with colobomas, Norrie's disease (see differential diagnosis of X-linked retinoschisis, in Chap. 3), cyclopia, and other conditions.[18]

Pathogenesis

Recent studies have suggested that apposition between the outer and inner layers of the optic cup is important for the sensory retina to develop properly.[18] If the sensory retina is separated from the retinal pigment epithelium in the embryo, retinal dysplasia may occur. This has been suggested because of the distribution of the dysplastic rosettes in cases of PHPV, colobomas, and related conditions. The possibility of a viral role exists, because retinal dysplasia has been produced experimentally by viral induction in the fetal lamb.[19]

REFERENCES

1. **Blodi FC:** Preretinal glial nodules in persistence and hyperplasia of the primary vitreous. Arch Ophthalmol 87:531–534, 1972
2. **Buettner H:** Congenital hypertrophy of the retinal pigment epithelium. Am J Ophthalmol 79:177–189, 1975
3. **Freeman HM:** Congenital retinal diseases. In Tasman WS (ed): Retinal Diseases in Children. New York, Harper & Row, 1971, pp 4–5
4. **Gass JDM:** Surgical excision of persistent hyperplastic primary vitreous. Arch Ophthalmol 83:163–168, 1970
5. **Jesberg DO, Schepens CL:** Retinal detachment associated with coloboma of the choroid. Arch Ophthalmol 65:163–173, 1961
6. **Mann I:** Congenital retinal fold. Br J Ophthalmol 19:641–658, 1935
7. **Manschot WA:** Persistent hyperplastic primary vitreous. Arch Ophthalmol 59:188–203, 1958
8. **Norris JL, Cleasley GW:** An unusual case of congenital hypertrophy of the retinal pigment epithelium. Arch Ophthalmol 94:1910–1911, 1976
9. **Pruett RC:** The pleomorphism and complications of posterior hyperplastic primary vitreous. Am J Ophthalmol 80:625–629, 1975

10. **Pruett RC, Schepens CL:** Posterior hyperplastic primary vitreous. Am J Ophthalmol 69:535–543, 1970

11. **Purcell JJ, Shields JA:** Hypertrophy with hyperpigmentation of the retinal pigment epithelium. Arch Ophthalmol 93:1122–1126, 1975

12. **Reese AB:** Persistence and hyperplasia of the primary vitreous: retrolental fibroplasia—two entities. Arch Ophthalmol 41:527–552, 1949

13. **Reese AB:** Persistent hyperplastic primary vitreous. The Jackson Memorial Lecture. Am J Ophthalmol 40:317–331, 1955

14. **Reese AB, Blodi FC:** Retinal dysplasia. Am J Ophthalmol 33:23–32, 1950

15. **Reese AB, Straatsma BR:** Retinal dysplasia. Am J Ophthalmol 45:199–211, 1958

16. **Shields JA:** Pathology of the vitreous. In Gitter KA (ed): Current Concepts of the Vitreous Including Vitrectomy. St. Louis, Mosby, 1976, pp 14–17

17. **Shields JA, Ts'o MOM:** Congenital grouped pigmentation of the retina. Histopathologic descriptions and report of a case. Arch Ophthalmol 93:1153–1155, 1975

18. **Silverstein AM, Osburn BI, Prendergast RA:** The pathogenesis of retinal dysplasia. Am J Ophthalmol 72:13–21, 1971

19. **Silverstein AM, Parshall CJ, Osburn BI, Prendergast RA:** An experimental viral induced dysplasia in the fetal lamb. Am J Ophthalmol 72:22–34, 1971

20. **Yanoff M, Fine BS:** Ocular Pathology. New York, Harper & Row, 1975, pp 29–59

5

Inflammatory Diseases

A number of inflammatory conditions may involve the peripheral fundus. Some of them tend to have a predilection for the peripheral retina, some for the uveal tract, and some for the sclera, while others produce the most reaction in the vitreous. Most inflammatory conditions, however, involve all of the structures to some degree.

As in other parts of the body, these inflammatory reactions may be due to bacterial, mycotic, viral, or parasitic organisms, or to hypersensitivity reactions. In the peripheral fundus, some of the most perplexing inflammations, both from a diagnostic and from a therapeutic point of view, are those which are presumed to be due to hypersensitivity reactions.

Many of the bacterial and fungal infections of the eye occur as part of a severe endophthalmitis following endogenous infection, ocular surgery, or ocular trauma. Such conditions will not be considered here. Rather, emphasis will be placed on those conditions which can selectively involve the structures of the peripheral fundus, often producing rather typical clinical features. These include "idiopathic" peripheral uveoretinitis, toxocariasis, sarcoidosis, nodular scleritis, toxoplasmosis, certain viral retinopathies, and sympathetic uveitis.

IDIOPATHIC PERIPHERAL UVEORETINITIS

This condition is a chronic inflammatory process involving the peripheral fundus, with a secondary cellular reaction in the vitreous. It has been the source of considerable confusion and controversy in the literature, particularly with regard to its terminology, etiology, and treatment.

Brockhurst and co-workers, reporting a large series of cases, preferred the term peripheral uveitis.[3] Later, the term pars planitis was introduced because the associated exudates are usually most concentrated in the pars plana region.[21] Other authorities prefer the term cyclitis, believing that the process is primarily an inflammation of the ciliary body.[8] Since it is now recognized that the inflammatory process involves the ciliary body, the peripheral choroid, and the peripheral retina, the name peripheral uveoretinitis would seem most accurate until further information regarding etiology is available (see also Etiology, below).

Clinical Features

Peripheral uveoretinitis may occur at any age but is most common and most severe in children and young adults. There appears to be no significant predilection for either sex. The condition is bilateral in about 95 percent of cases, and the symptoms are variable, ranging from mild to severe.

The ocular findings include decreased visual acuity, normal or slightly decreased intraocular pressure, a few small nongranulomatous keratic precipitates, and a slight aqueous flare. The most consistent finding, which is mandatory for the clinical diagnosis, is a biomicroscopic demonstration of flare and cells in the anterior vitreous. Ophthalmoscopy with scleral depression often demonstrates white exudates in the region of the vitreous base (Fig. 5-1) and in the pars plana region. The exudates may be located in any quadrant but are most pronounced inferiorly.

The peripheral retinal vessels, particularly the veins, may show dilatation and occasional perivascular exudates. Cystoid maculopathy, which may cause moderate visual loss, is a frequent associated finding. Fluorescein angiography often demonstrates generalized leakage from the retinal vessels and late staining of the cystoid spaces in the fovea.

The disease is chronic and may smolder for years, with exacerbations and remissions but with a gradual downhill course. With time, peripheral anterior synechiae, posterior subcapsular cataract, and vitreous fibrosis may occur. As the vitreous inflammation becomes more organized, traction on the peripheral retina may lead to peripheral retinoschisis and retinal detachment, either with or without a retinal hole. The eventual result may be blindness from glaucoma, cataract, or band keratopathy. The two most common complications leading to visual loss are cataract and macular degeneration.[19]

Pathology

The pathology of idiopathic peripheral uveoretinitis has been studied in only a few cases and no specific inflammatory agent has been found. However, certain more specific inflammatory conditions, such as sacroidosis and toxocariasis, produce a similar clinical picture that has been documented histologically. The main pathologic changes include a chronic nongranulomatous retinal periphlebitis and chronic inflammatory cells in the vitreous. There

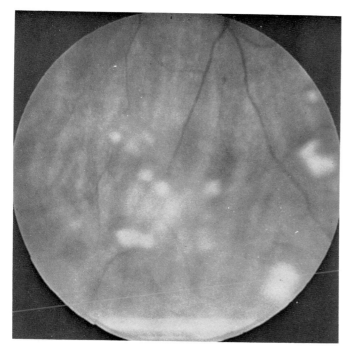

FIG. 5-1. White exudates in the inferior vitreous of a patient with peripheral uveoretinitis.

FIG. 5-2. Exudate in the region of the vitreous base in a patient with peripheral uveoretinitis. The ciliary epithelium is below. (AFIP accession no. 1255679) (Hematoxylin-eosin stain; ×55)

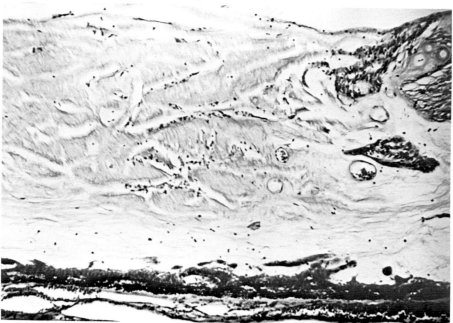

may be a massive amount of rather homogeneous eosinophilic exudate in the peripheral vitreous (Fig. 5-2). The inflammatory infiltrate appears to leave the uveal tract relatively uninvolved.

Etiology

The etiology of peripheral uveoretinitis is unknown, although many authorities believe that it represents a peculiar hypersensitivity reaction to the small peripheral retinal vessels. If this is the case, perhaps the term peripheral retinal vasculitis would be a more accurate name. Although, as mentioned, no specific etiological factor can be incriminated in most cases, certain well-recognized entities have been documented to produce a similar clinical and histologic picture. These entities are all-important in the differential diagnosis of this condition.

Differential Diagnosis

The differential diagnosis of idiopathic peripheral uveoretinitis includes sarcoidosis, *Toxocara* endophthalmitis, toxoplasmosis, and other causes of intraocular inflammation. Most of these are discussed in detail later in this chapter; clinical and laboratory findings should aid in the differentiation. Retinoblastoma also may resemble peripheral uveoretinitis; their differentiation is discussed in Chapter 7.

Treatment

Mild cases may be managed with topical corticosteroids. In more severe cases with macular edema, systemic or locally injected corticosteroids may be necessary. In advanced cases with complications, immunosuppressive agents may be useful.

   Some authorities have advocated the use of cryotherapy in the management of peripheral uveoretinitis.[1] Eradication of the small peripheral retinal vessels by this technique may remove the vascular focus for the antigen-antibody reaction which is thought to lead to the inflammation.[15]

NEMATODE ENDOPHTHALMITIS

Nematode endophthalmitis, most commonly due to ocular infestation with the second-stage larva of the dog roundworm, *Toxocara canis*, is recognized as a frequent cause of intraocular inflammation. It may occur in a variety of forms, such as an isolated chorioretinal granuloma in the posterior pole, or peculiar pigmented "tracks" beneath the retina due to migration of the para-

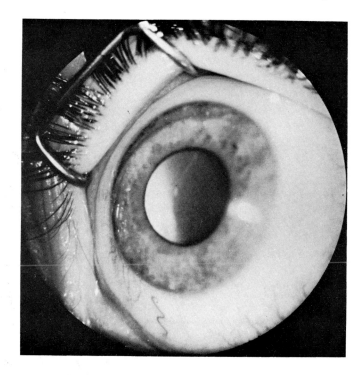

FIG. 5-3. Inflammatory reaction in the peripheral vitreous overlying a nematode granuloma.

site. Most commonly, however, the condition involves the peripheral fundus and produces an isolated granuloma with severe vitreous traction.

Clinical Features

The patient usually presents to the ophthalmologist during the first 3 to 6 years of life. Typically, on routine school examination the child is discovered to have poor vision in the involved eye. The condition is almost always unilateral and shows no predisposition for either sex or race.

The history is often unremarkable, but there is usually previous contact with puppies. The child may have had a history of fever of unknown origin about 1 to 2 years prior to the discovery of the ocular problem. This may indicate previous visceral larva migrans. If there was associated hepatosplenomegaly and eosinophilia, this further suggests that the ocular lesion may be due to *Toxocara*.

The general physical findings are usually normal and there is usually no eosinophilia when the child presents to the ophthalmologist. Ocular examination (Fig. 5-3) reveals signs of anterior uveitis with a hazy anterior vitreous. The peripheral fundus will show an elevated hazy white mass that may be mistaken for retinoblastoma (see in Chap. 7). The lesion may shrink, causing

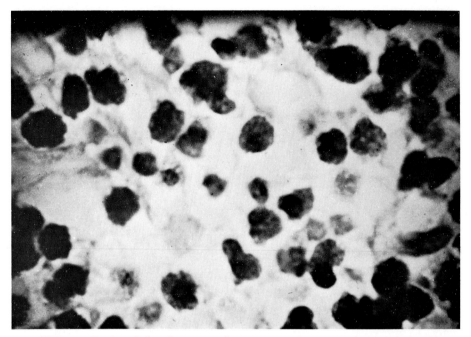

FIG. 5-4. Eosinophilic abscess in the vitreous of a patient with nematode endophthalmitis. (Hematoxylin-eosin stain; ×300)

dragging of the retina and producing a retinal fold. Progression to vitreous traction bands, retinal detachment, cyclitic membrane, cataract, secondary glaucoma, and eventually phthisis bulbi comprise the natural course of the disease.

Histopathology

Some eyes with nematode and endophthalmitis have been enucleated for suspected retinoblastoma, and other eyes because of intractable glaucoma due to iris bombé or rubeosis iridis. Sections usually reveal a total retinal detachment with subretinal exudation. The peripheral retina and vitreous may contain an abscess composed of eosinophils (Fig. 5-4). Serial sections may reveal a well-preserved larva, or its necrotic remnants, within the area of inflammation (Fig. 5-5).

Diagnostic Techniques

Certain laboratory tests are helpful in the diagnosis, although none is absolutely specific. Skin tests have been of limited value because of cross reactions with Ascaris. The enzyme-linked immunosorbent assay (ELISA test) has shown promise as a diagnostic test for ocular toxocariasis.[13, 16] The demonstra-

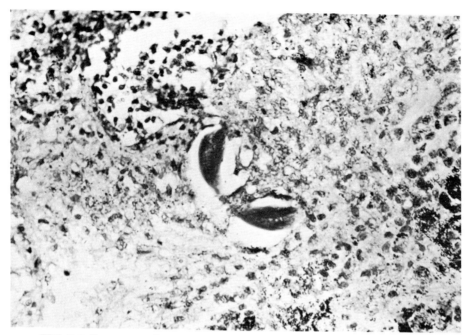

FIG. 5-5. Remnants of a nematode larva within a necrotic abscess of the retina. (Hematoxylin-eosin stain; ×150)

tion of eosinophils in aspirated vitreous or aqueous may further substantiate the diagnosis.[17] Negative tests for aqueous enzymes such as lactate dehydrogenase (LDH) and phosphoglucose isomerase (PGI) by helping to exclude the diagnosis of retinoblastoma, may lend support to the diagnosis of toxocariasis.[5]

Pathogenesis

Ocular toxocariasis occurs in patients previously infested with visceral larva migrans. The ova are probably ingested by eating dirt or by close contact with puppies. The larvae hatch in the intestine, and the second-stage larva has the ability to reach the bloodstream and migrate to many organs, including the eye, where granulomas may develop.

Treatment

In many cases, the ocular lesion responds poorly to treatment, and severe complications are inevitable. Specific drugs for roundworms are only questionably effective. If the inflammatory granuloma is discovered early enough, the one or more injections of corticosteroids subconjunctivally in the quad-

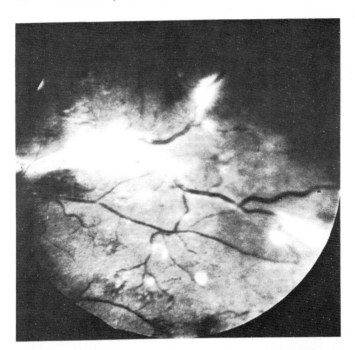

FIG. 5-6. Fundus photograph of retinal periphlebitis in a patient with sarcoidosis.

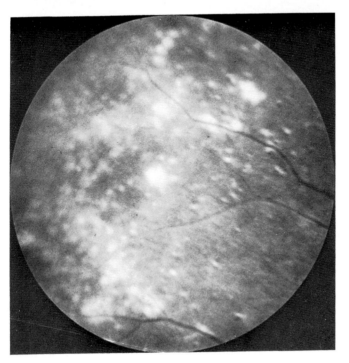

FIG. 5-7. Fundus photograph showing vitreous and retinal opacities in a patient with sarcoidosis.

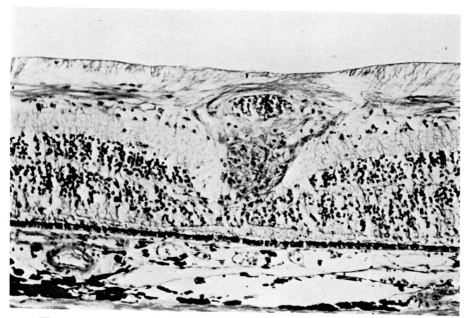

FIG. 5-8. Sarcoid granuloma adjacent to a retinal blood vessel. (AFIP accession no. 1378625) (Hematoxylin-eosin stain; ×145)

rant of the lesion may quiet the inflammatory process and minimize the complications.[17]

SARCOIDOSIS

Sarcoidosis (see also in Chap. 6) is a disease of unknown etiology characterized by fever, lymphadenopathy, arthritis, and numerous central nervous system symptoms. Any part of the eye or adnexa may be involved with sarcoidosis.[10]

Clinical Features

The changes in the peripheral fundus that can occur in sarcoidosis include retinal periphlebitis (Fig. 5-6), retinal hemorrhages, subretinal granulomas, vitreous opacities (Fig. 5-7), and exudates in the pars plana which resemble those of idiopathic peripheral uveoretinitis.[9] The retinal periphlebitis may be so intense that it produces typical "candle-wax drippings." Retinal involvement is usually associated with some degree of concurrent central nervous system involvement.

Pathology

Histopathologically, sarcoidosis of the peripheral fundus is characterized by subretinal or intraretinal granulomas (Fig. 5-8), retinal periphlebitis, and cells

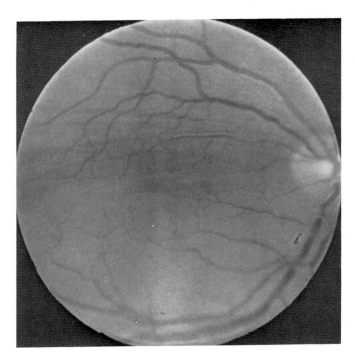

FIG. 5-9. Fundus photo-graph of posterior sclerit showing elevated retina below the macula, with a serous retinal detachmen and choroidal folds.

in the vitreous. The subretinal granulomas are small, noncaseating lesions containing epithelioid cells and are located immediately beneath the retinal pigment epithelium. In contrast to the Dalen-Fuchs nodules of sympathetic uveitis (see below), they are said to break through the retinal pigment epithelium, producing inflammation of the sensory retina.

There is a cuff of lymphocytic infiltration along the retinal veins, caus-ing the perivasculitis seen clinically. The lymphocytes may break into the vitreous, which could explain the vitreous opacities seen clinically.

Diagnosis

The diagnosis of sarcoidosis is based on the ocular findings previously de-scribed, in addition to a general physical examination and laboratory tests. These should include x-rays of the lungs and joints, serum protein elec-trophoresis, and perhaps a Kveim skin test. The techniques and normal values of the procedures are described in the literature.[9]

Sarcoidosis is much more common in blacks than in whites and should be considered in the differential diagnosis of all cases of posterior segment inflammation in black patients.

Treatment

There is no specific therapy for ocular sarcoidosis. Once the diagnosis is established, corticosteroids appear to be the treatment of choice. In cases with retinal involvement they may be given by either periocular injection or oral administration. The dose should vary with the severity of the disease.

NODULAR SCLERITIS

Nodular scleritis is a rather uncommon inflammatory condition which primarily involves the sclera but secondarily affects the overlying uveal tract, producing sclerouveitis. The anterior type involves the ciliary region and often occurs in patients with rheumatoid arthritis, whereas the posterior type is frequently seen in patients with no known systemic disease. The anterior type can usually be seen on external ocular examination, while the posterior type is only seen on fundus examination.

Clinical Features

The patient with nodular posterior scleritis is often systemically well. There may be a history of recurrent bouts of diffuse anterior scleritis. Anterior segment examination is otherwise normal.

Fundus examination reveals a nonpigmented placoid to oval mass which is often the same color as the background fundus.[2] The lesion may occur near the equator, but is more commonly posterior. It often has an associated retinal detachment with yellowish white particles in the subretinal space. Choroidal folds are frequently present in a pattern which is concentric to the margins of the lesion (Fig. 5-9).

Fluorescein angiography shows splotchy foci of hyperfluorescence which gradually become larger and less distinct in the late angiograms. Ultrasonography shows an oval-shaped mass with high internal reflectivity. There may be an area without orbital echoes immediately behind the sclera, similar to that seen with orbital inflammation of any cause.

Pathology

Histologic examination reveals an oval-shaped or diffuse thickening of the sclera that corresponds to the lesion seen clinically. It results from disruption of the normal scleral architecture, which is replaced by chronic inflammatory cells. The inflammation may be granulomatous or nongranulomatous. The choroid may be thickened, and a serous retinal detachment is often present (Fig. 5-10).

Differential Diagnosis

The differential diagnosis of nodular scleritis includes both intraocular and orbital tumors. The three most common ocular tumors to be considered include amelanotic melanoma, choroidal hemangioma, and tumor metastatic to the choroid (see Malignant Melanoma, in Chap. 7). The inflammatory signs

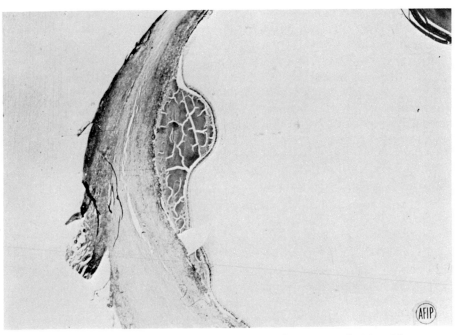

FIG. 5-10. Low-power photomicrograph of nongranulomatous scleritis with an overlying serous retinal detachment. (Hematoxylin-eosin stain; ×25)

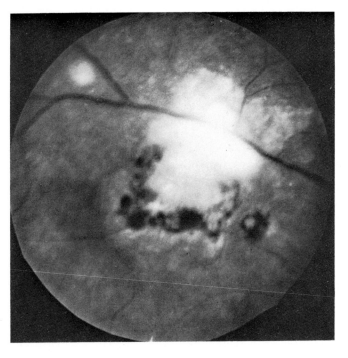

FIG. 5-11. Fundus photograph showing acu| toxoplasmic retinochoroi(adjacent to a chronic inac lesion.

that are associated with scleritis should be helpful. Also, the typical concentric choroidal folds are common with scleritis and extremely rare with choroidal tumors, while ultrasonography shows signs of retrobulbar inflammation in cases of scleritis, a finding rarely observed with intraocular tumors.[2]

Orbital lesions (e.g., mucoceles, hemangiomas, or dermoids) may press on the globe and simulate scleritis. They usually slide along the sclera with movements of the eye, whereas nodular scleritis moves with the globe. Ultrasonography and computerized axial tomography should be helpful in the differentiation.

Treatment

Posterior nodular scleritis, like anterior scleritis, is responsive to treatment with corticosteroids. These may be given by periocular injection in the quadrant of the lesion or they may be given systemically.

TOXOPLASMOSIS

Toxoplasmosis, caused by the protozoon *Toxoplasma gondii,* can be either congenital or acquired after birth. It is most commonly associated with lesions in the posterior pole, but peripheral lesions are also encountered. Both the congenital and the acquired forms may involve the peripheral fundus. The pathogenesis and basic aspects of this disease are well described in the literature.[14]

Clinical Features

In the acute stage, there is a fluffy white lesion of the retina which is associated with an inflammatory reaction in the overlying vitreous (Fig. 5-11). There may be sheathing of the retinal vessels. There is often a nonspecific inflammatory reaction in the anterior chamber, with flare and cells in the aqueous and granulomatous keratic precipitates. Pigmented chorioretinal scars, called satellite lesions, are usually present adjacent to the active inflammatory process.

In the chronic or inactive stage, there is a well delineated, depressed, pigmented chorioretinal scar. Signs of anterior segment inflammation are usually lacking.

Pathology

Toxoplasmosis is classically described as a segmental panophthalmitis. There is granulomatous scleritis, choroiditis, and a necrotizing coagulative retinitis (Fig. 5-12). The *Toxoplasma* organisms are usually confined to the sensory retina (Fig. 5-13).

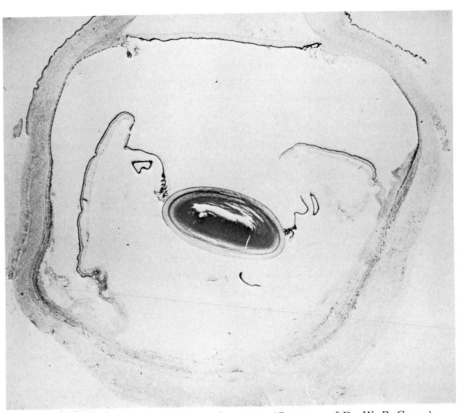

FIG. 5-12. Severe congenital toxoplasmosis. (Courtesy of Dr. W. R. Green)

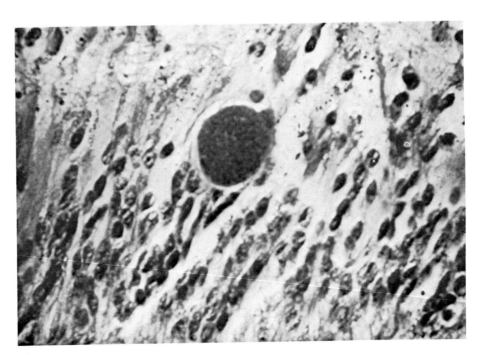

Diagnosis

The diagnosis of toxoplasmosis is based on the recognition of the typical clinical features, in conjunction with laboratory tests. A history of contact with cats or of ingesting raw meat will help lead to the correct diagnosis of the acquired form.

Laboratory studies include the older Sabin-Feldman dye test and the more commonly employed immunofluorescent antibody test. Most larger laboratories are equipped to perform these procedures. If ocular or lymph node tissue is available, its injection into purebred mice should reproduce the disease and thus establish the diagnosis.[11]

Treatment

The treatment of toxoplasmosis depends on the extent of the disease. If the lesion is in the peripheral retina and not affecting vision, many authorities would advocate not treating it. If visual acuity is decreased or threatened, therapy with pyrimethamine and a sulfonamide is recommended.[12] A newer drug, clindamycin, is presently being used in some cases.

VIRAL RETINOPATHIES

A number of viral diseases are now known to involve the ocular fundus. Some occur as opportunistic disease in debilitated patients, while others occur in healthy individuals. There is no specific treatment for most viral retinopathies.

CYTOMEGALOVIRUS RETINITIS

Although cytomegalovirus has been known to produce a systemic syndrome in infants, it has more recently been recognized as the cause of a severe retinitis in adults who are debilitated or immunosuppressed.[4, 19] Cytomegalovirus retinitis is therefore more likely to occur in cancer patients who are taking chemotherapy or corticosteroids, or in patients who have had renal or other organ transplants and are being managed with immunosuppressive drugs.

Clinically, the patient presents with a variably sized area of retinal necrosis characterized by irregular thickening of the retina, with focal hemorrhages that may be superficial or deep (Fig. 5-14). There is frequently a nonspecific inflammatory reaction in the anterior segment.

Histologically, there is extensive retinal necrosis with a chronic in-

---

FIG. **5-13.** *Toxoplasma* cyst in the retina. (AFIP accession no. 1180883) (Hematoxylin-eosin stain; ×400)

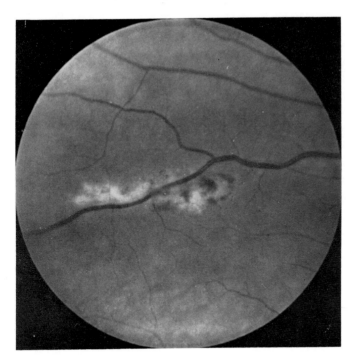

FIG. 5-14. Fundus photograph showing focal area of hemorrhagic necro of the retina in a patient w cytomegalic inclusion retinitis. The patient had systemic lymphoma.

FIG. 5-15. Low-power photomicrograph of retinal necrosis secondary to cytomegalic inclusion disease. (AFIP accession no. 1108704) (Hematoxylin-eosin stain; ×10)

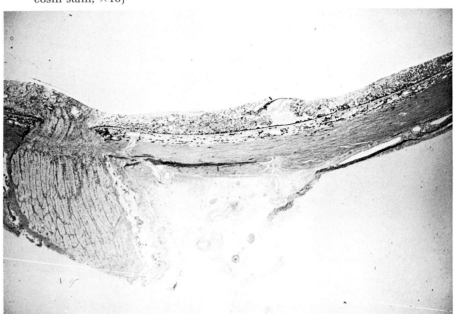

flammatory cell infiltrate (Fig. 5-15). Typical large cells with basophilic intra-nuclear inclusions can be seen in the involved areas of the retina.

Treatment involves discontinuing any immunosuppresive drugs, if possible. Immunostimulant substances, such as transfer factor, are being used experimentally.

SUBACUTE SCLEROSING PANENCEPHALITIS

It has recently been recognized that the slow virus of measles which produces subacute sclerosing panencephalitis (SSPE, Dawson's encephalitis) may affect the eye as well as the brain. The precise pathogenesis is uncertain, but the ophthalmic clinical and pathologic features have been described.[6, 7]

Clinically, the condition usually occurs in young children between 6 and 12 years of age. They develop a progressive neurologic syndrome with the signs and symptoms of encephalitis. The involved retina may show a serous detachment of the fovea, followed by a dry pigmentary maculopathy. The peripheral retina shows white or yellow nodules which gradually resolve to form pigmentary scars (Fig. 5-16).

Pathologically, there is retinal necrosis with degeneration of the retinal pigment epithelium. Particles compatible with the paramyxovirus of measles have been recognized in the retina.[6]

RUBELLA

The widespread ocular manifestations of congenital rubella (see Rubella Retinopathy in Chap. 3) are now well known.[22] The retina may show diffuse mottled pigmentary involvement (Fig. 5-17; see also Fig. 3-25 in Chap. 3). The history of maternal rubella should aid in the diagnosis. Pathologically, there are alterations in the retinal pigment epithelium which correlate with the clinical features (Fig. 5-18).

HERPES SIMPLEX RETINITIS

Recent studies have shown that some cases of peripheral fundus inflammation may be due to invasion of the retina by herpes simplex virus. This virus produces a clinical picture similar to that of the other types of viral retinitis. The retinitis may be associated with a rather severe or subclinical encephalitis.

SYMPATHETIC UVEITIS

Clinical Features

The clinical features of sympathetic uveitis are well known. It usually follows a penetrating injury to the globe, in the region of the ciliary body, that has

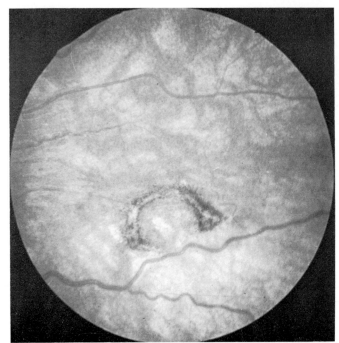

FIG. 5-16. Fundus photograph of a fundus scar secondary to retinal infiltration in a patient with subacute sclerosing panencephalitis (SSPE).

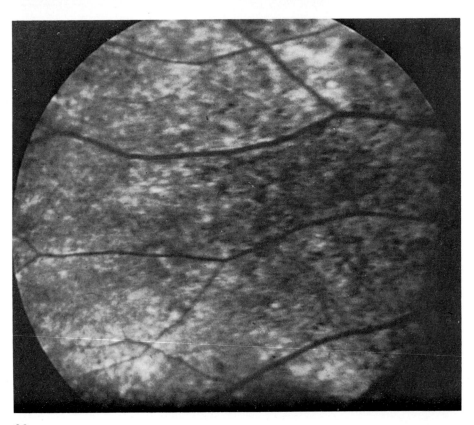

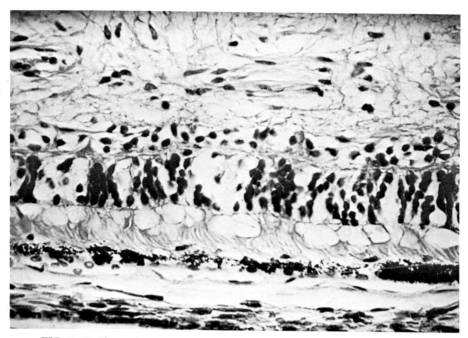

FIG. 5-18. The retina in a patient with rubella retinopathy. Note the alterations in the retinal pigment epithelium (below). (AFIP accession no. 997770) (Hematoxylin-eosin stain; ×250)

caused the prolapse or loss of uveal tissue. The injured eye shows a rather severe inflammatory reaction, with anterior granulomatous uveitis. Between 10 and 14 days after the injury, the patient may show cells in the retrolental space of the opposite eye, followed by a frank granulomatous uveitis. The peripheral fundus may show yellowish white subretinal nodules (Dalen-Fuchs nodules). Sympathetic uveitis is believed to be due to a hypersensitivity reaction to the injured uveal tissue.

Pathology

Pathologically, the injured eye and the sympathizing eye show a severe granulomatous reaction, with giant cells and pigment phagocytosis. The entire uveal tract may exhibit a diffuse infiltration, with chronic inflammatory cells which produce marked choroidal thickening with sparing of the choriocapillaris (Fig. 5-19). Typical Dalen-Fuchs nodules may be present beneath the retinal pigment epithelium (Fig. 5-20); they are believed to represent focal epithelioid granulomas.

⟵————FIG. 5-17. Fundus photograph of pigment alterations in a patient with rubella retinopathy.

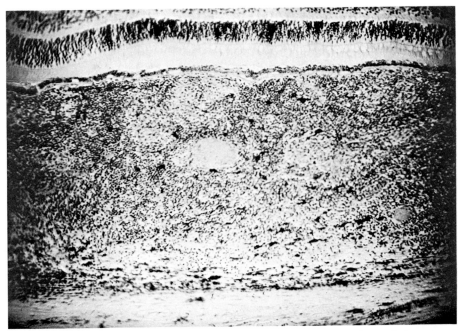

FIG. 5-19. Sympathetic uveitis showing thickening of the choroid due to infiltration by chronic inflammatory cells. (Hematoxylin-eosin stain; ×75)

FIG. 5-20. Dalen-Fuchs nodule beneath the pigment epithelium in an eye with sympathetic uveitis. (AFIP accession no. 909318) (Hematoxylin-eosin stain; ×200)

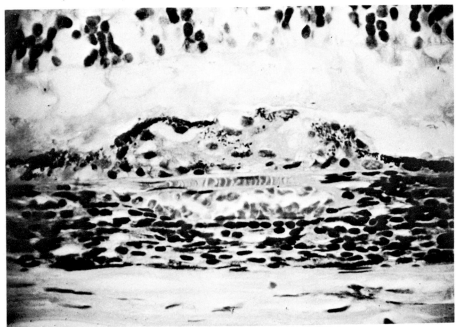

Treatment

Sympathetic uveitis is best treated prophylactically, by enucleation of the traumatized eye prior to involvement of the sympathizing eye. This is acceptable if the traumatized eye has no possibility of useful vision. If the eye has useful vision, however, it may sometimes be preferable to treat with systemic or topical corticosteroids alone. Whether the injured eye should be enucleated if the second eye becomes involved is questionable. When the disease is active in the second eye, systemic, periocular, and topical corticosteroids should be given in the minimal amount necessary to control the symptoms, in order to prevent complications of the uveitis.

REFERENCES

1. **Aaberg TM, Cesarz TJ, Flickinger RR:** Treatment of peripheral uveoretinitis by cryotherapy. Am J Ophthalmol 75:685–688, 1973
2. **Benson WE, Shields JA, Tasman WS, Crandall AS:** Nodular posterior scleritis. Arch Ophthalmol 97:1482–1486, 1979
3. **Brockhurst RJ, Schepens CL, Okamura ID:** Peripheral uveitis. Clinical description, complications and differential diagnosis. Am J Ophthalmol 49:1257–1266, 1960
4. **DeVenecia G, Rhein GMZ, Pratt MV, Kisken W:** Cytomegalic inclusion retinitis in an adult. Arch Ophthalmol 86:44–57, 1971
5. **Felberg NT, McFall R, Shields JA:** Aqueous humor enzyme patterns in retinoblastoma. Invest Ophthalmol 16:1039–1046, 1977
6. **Font RL, Jenis EH, Tuck KD:** Measles maculopathy associated with subacute sclerosing panencephalitis. Arch Pathol Lab Med 96:168–174, 1973
7. **Hiatt RL, Grizzard HT, McNeer P, Jabbour JT:** Ophthalmologic manifestations of subacute sclerosing panencephalitis (Dawson's disease). Trans Am Acad Ophthalmol Otolaryngol 75:344–350, 1971
8. **Hogan MJ, Kimura SJ:** Cyclitis and peripheral chorioretinitis. Arch Ophthalmol 66:667–677, 1961
9. **Letocha CE, Shields JA, Goldberg RE:** Retinal changes in sarcoidosis. Can J Ophthalmol 10:184–192, 1975
10. **Maumenee AE, Zimmerman LE:** Ocular aspects of sarcoidosis. Am Rev Resp Dis 84(5)Pt 2:38–44, 1961
11. **Michelson JB, Shields JA, McDonald PR, Manko MM, Abraham AA, Federman JL:** Retinitis secondary to acquired systemic toxoplasmosis with isolation of the parasite. Am J Ophthalmol 86:548–552, 1978
12. **O'Connor GR:** Manifestations and management of ocular toxoplasmosis. Bull NY Acad Med 50:192–210, 1974
13. **Pollard ZF, Jarrett WH, Hagler WS, Allain DS, Schantz PM:** ELISA for diagnosis of ocular toxocariasis. Ophthalmology (in press)
14. **Schlaegel TF:** Essentials of Uveitis. Boston, Little, Brown, 1969, pp 181–203
15. **Schlaegel TF:** Miscellaneous uveitis syndromes. In Duane TD (ed): Clinical Ophthalmology, Vol 4. Hagerstown, Harper & Row, 1976
16. **Shields JA, Felberg, NT, Federman JL:** Discussion of ELISA for the diagnosis of ocular toxocariasis. Ophthalmology (in press)
17. **Shields JA, Lerner HA, Felberg NT:** Aqueous cytology and enzymes in nematode endophthalmitis. Am J Ophthalmol 84:319–322, 1977
18. **Smith ME, Zimmerman LE, Harley RD:** Ocular involvement in congenital cytomegalic inclusion disease. Arch Ophthalmol 76:696–699, 1966
19. **Smith RE, Godfrey WA, Kimura SJ:** Chronic cyclitis. I. Course and visual prognosis. Trans Am Acad Ophthalmol Otolaryngol 77:760–768, 1973
20. **Tate GW, Martin RG:** Clindamycin in the treatment of human ocular toxoplasmosis. Can J Ophthalmol 12:188–195, 1977
21. **Welch RB, Maumenee AE, Wahlen HE:** Peripheral posterior segment inflammation, vitreous opacities, and edema of the posterior pole. Pars planitis. Arch Ophthalmol 64:540–549, 1960
22. **Zimmerman LE:** Histopathologic basis for ocular manifestations of congenital rubella syndrome. Am J Ophthalmol 65:837–862, 1968

6

Vascular Abnormalities

DIABETES MELLITUS

Diabetes mellitus is a genetically determined disorder of metabolism which in its fully developed clinical expression is characterized by fasting hyperglycemia, arteriosclerotic and microangiopathic vascular disease, and neuropathy. The progression of diabetes from one stage to the next may occur very slowly over many years or may be rapid or even explosive. Diagnosis depends upon the proper use and interpretation of laboratory procedures.

Hereditary Aspects and Incidence

It is estimated that there are about ten million diabetics or potential diabetics in the United States at the present time, an incidence of 1 in 20, or 5 percent of the population. Of all diabetics, 8 percent are under the age of 25 when the diagnosis is made. An additional 22 percent of patients are diagnosed between the ages of 25 and 44, 50 percent between the ages of 45 and 64, and 20 percent after the age of 65. Overall, 70 percent of diabetics are 45 years old or older.

Evidence for the importance of hereditary factors in the evolution of diabetes is demonstrated by the high concordance rate among monozygotic twins as compared to dizygotic twins. Inheritance of diabetes as estimated from sibling correlations has been found to be 70 to 80 percent among diabetic children under 10 years of age and 30 to 40 percent in diabetics 50 years old and older. In addition, when there is a family history of diabetes, it may be estimated that 1 percent of diabetics have three generations involved, 17 percent have diabetic mothers, 8 percent have diabetic fathers, and 25 percent of diabetics with siblings have another sibling who is affected.

DIABETIC RETINOPATHY

Incidence

A major complication of diabetes is blindness. The overall incidence of diabetic retinopathy in the diabetic population in 1921, according to Wagner and Wilder, was about 8.3 percent.[53] By 1972, Cullen reported diabetic retinopathy as responsible for 41 percent of all cases of blindness in males and 58 percent in females.[12] In 1975, Kahn and Bradley identified diabetic retinopathy as the cause of blindness in 24 percent of patients who have lost their sight.[29] In general, it may also be assumed that approximately 50 percent of all diabetics will have retinopathy at the time their diabetes is diagnosed. However, Oakley et al. found that 30 percent of patients with diabetes of 40 years' duration or more were still unaffected by retinopathy.[39]

The incidence of diabetic retinopathy varies with age at the time of diagnosis and with duration of the disease. For example, Burdett, Caird, and Draper[6] in 1968 found that 73 percent of diabetics who had been diagnosed before the age of 30 had significant retinopathy after 15 years' duration of the disease. On the other hand, 59 percent of those diagnosed as diabetic after the age of 60 had significant retinopathy after 15 years' duration of the disease. Similar figures were reported in 1975 by Kahn and Bradley, who also found a high incidence of retinopathy after 15 years' duration of the disease in younger diabetics than in those who were diagnosed after the age of 65.[29] It does appear, therefore, that the prevalence of retinopathy is strongly associated with the duration of the disease. It also appears that the prevalence of retinopathy may be more strongly related to duration of disease in women than in men, and that females are more frequently affected than males (in a ratio of 3:2) and black females more often than white females.

In 1972, Cullen found the overall incidence of proliferative diabetic retinopathy to be 4.4 percent in a group of 5147 diabetics.[12] The incidence of this form of retinopathy was higher in insulin-dependent diabetics than in non-insulin-dependent diabetics.

Thus, of the diseases which affect the retinal vasculature, the one that is probably most devastating to sight is diabetes mellitus. Diabetic retinopathy is becoming an ever-increasing cause of legal blindness in the United States, as the incidence of cases continues to increase at an annual rate of about 6 percent.

Classification of Diabetic Retinopathy

Diabetes-related disorders of sight can be classified into two large categories: (1) the so-called background diabetic retinopathy and (2) proliferative diabetic retinopathy.

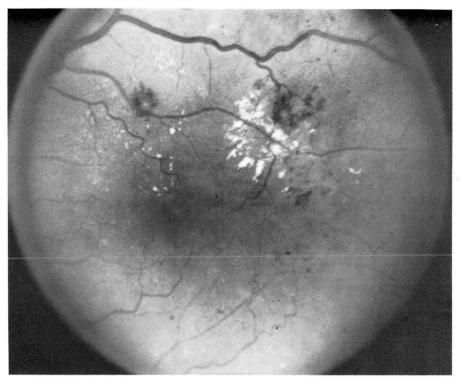

FIG. 6-1. Background diabetic retinopathy with retinal hemorrhages and exudates in the posterior pole.

Background diabetic retinopathy primarily affects the posterior pole and is intraretinal: microaneurysms and retinal hemorrhages, exudation, and macular edema are apparent (Fig. 6-1). Although it may lead to legal blindness, it does not result in retinal detachment or severe vitreous hemorrhage which could prevent ambulation. By contrast, proliferative diabetic retinopathy is characterized by extraretinal proliferation of vessels, and is much more severe, resulting at times in retinal breaks and detachments, and intractable vitreous hemorrhage.

Often the proliferative retinopathy is heralded by a more florid and advanced phase of background diabetic retinopathy referred to as preproliferative retinopathy. The ophthalmoscopic signs consist of soft exudates (cotton-wool spots), venous beading, and intraretinal microvascular abnormalities. Fluorescein angiography has shown that the soft exudates, once thought to be indicative of associated hypertension, actually correspond to focal areas of capillary nonperfusion that produce an infarct, with swelling of the nerve fiber layer of the retina. These changes occur frequently in normotensive patients as well as hypertensive patients. Venous beading consists of irregular, sausage-shaped changes in the appearance of the retinal veins. Intraretinal microvascular abnormalities are dilated capillary shunt vessels in the retina. These frequently develop around focal areas of capillary nonperfu-

sion. Fluorescein angiography provides another sign of preproliferative retinopathy, namely, large and extensive areas of capillary closure. This is a
feature common to other proliferative retinopathies as well, notably branch
vein occlusion and retrolental fibroplasia.

The developmental stages of proliferative diabetic retinopathy have
been described by Dobree.[15] Proliferative lesions in the diabetic retina often
begin as a collection of fine, naked vessels, the intraretinal microvascular
abnormalities already referred to (Stage 1) (Fig. 6-2). Later, extraretinal new
vessels develop on the retina or on the optic nerve head (Fig. 6-3). These
progress through a stage of vascular proliferation with connective tissue
formation (Stage 2). In Stage 2, the neovascular proliferations, which occur
secondary to capillary obliteration, frequently grow into or towards the zone
of retinal ischemia. In some cases there is a terminating stage (Stage 3),
characterized by regression of the vascular systems with contracture of the
connective tissue components, development of retinovitreal bands, thickening of the posterior vitreous face, and the appearance of retinoschisis, retinal
detachments, and retinal holes.

Of particular importance, as Dobree has emphasized, is the significance
of vitreous traction as a factor in the natural history of proliferative diabetic
retinopathy. Davis et al.[13] also aptly stressed the role of the contracting
vitreous in the production of vitreous hemorrhage, retinal breaks, and retinal

FIG. 6-2. Juvenile diabetic with hemorrhages in the posterior pole and
intraretinal microvascular abnormalities along the superior temporal vessels
(*arrow*). The intraretinal microvascular abnormalities do not leak on fluorescein
angiography and are intraretinal, in contrast to neovascularization, which is on
the surface of the retina.

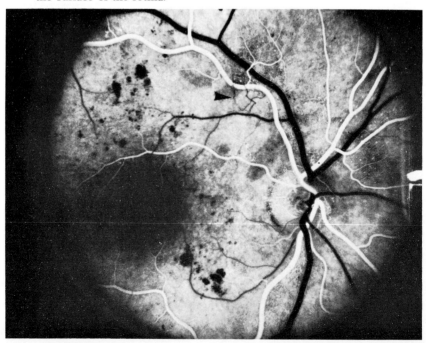

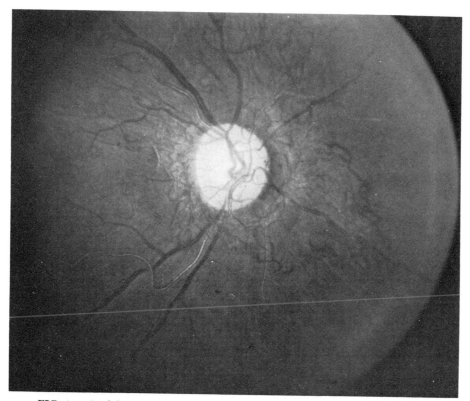

FIG. 6-3. Proliferative diabetic retinopathy: Neovascularization on the disc.

detachments. In their view, retinal detachment and the presence of neovascular tissue in the vitreous cavity are caused not so much by an active anterior growth of neovascular tissue as by a more passive effect of contracting vitreous which has become adherent to the neovascular tissue and retina. Evidence from fluorescein angiography seems to support this view, since patients who have had vitrectomies show much less leakage from neovascular areas postoperatively than they did preoperatively. Retinoschisis and retinal holes also appear to develop as a result of vitreous traction.

In a further study of the course of proliferative diabetic retinopathy, McMeel[35] classified in detail the advanced fibrotic stages. He noted two common types of fibrotic tissues, fibrovascular proliferative tissue and avascular proliferative tissue, and an infrequent iatrogenic type arising at the borders of photocoagulation scars. He most frequently observed the fibrovascular variety, which he found in association with vessels extending into the vitreous chamber or with abnormal new vessels on the surface of the retina or disc. He further divided the avascular variety into three types: (1) a direct extension from the fibrovascular variety; (2) vitreous membranes unassociated with fibrovascular tissue (vitreoretinal ridges); and (3) preretinal membranes, also known as preretinal organization or thickening of the posterior hyaloid face. Traction on the retina was observed with all forms of fibrotic proliferations except the thickened posterior hyaloid face and the iatrogenic type.

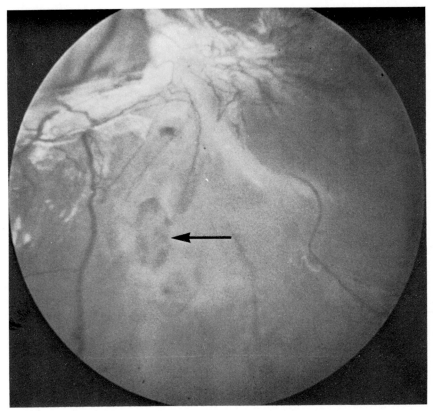

FIG. 6-4. Proliferative retinopathy in a juvenile diabetic, showing retinal detachment and retinal break formation (*arrow*) near the area of proliferans.

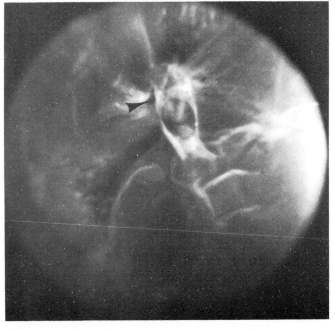

FIG. 6-5. Equator-plus (wide-angle) photograph of diabetic tractional retinal detachment with hole (*arrow*) in the posterior j

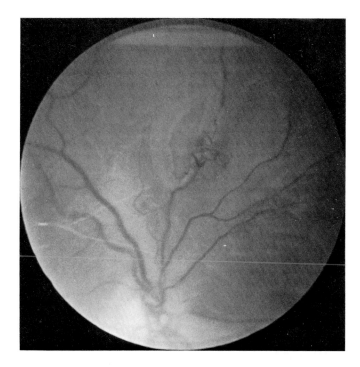

FIG. 6-6. Large break (*arrow*) near an area of neovascularization in a patient with proliferative diabetic retinopathy.

Traction Retinal Detachments

McMeel[35] and Tasman[47] also distinguished between traction detachments, which were not caused by retinal breaks (nonrhegmatogenous), and detachments directly caused by retinal breaks (rhegmatogenous). In McMeel's series of diabetic retinal detachment,[35] about 75 percent were nonrhegmatogenous (traction variety), approximately 20 percent were rhegmatogenous, and the remainder were not classified.

Characteristics of the nonrhegmatogenous detachments in proliferative diabetic retinopathy included the following: (1) an elevation of the retina that was confined to the posterior fundus and infrequently extending more than two-thirds of the distance to the equator; (2) a taut retina with a shiny surface; (3) frequently observed demarcation lines, indicating that extension of the detachment was common; and (4) no shifting of subretinal fluid or mobility of the retina. In a few cases, both McMeel and Tasman noted a spontaneous decrease in the extent of the traction detachment.

By contrast, in proliferative diabetic retinopathy the borders of a rhegmatogenous detachment usually extend to the ora serrata; the retinal surface is dull, grayish, and undulates because of the retinal mobility and some shifting of subretinal fluid. Retinal breaks are usually in the posterior pole near areas of fibrovascular change (Fig. 6-4, 6-5, and 6-6). The breaks are oval in shape and appear to be more the result of tangential traction from the proliferative tissue than vitreous traction. Determining the location of retinal holes may be complicated by many factors, particularly poor dilation of the pupil, lens opacity, increased vitreous turbidity, vitreous hemorrhage, intraretinal hemorrhage, and obscuration of the breaks by overlying proliferative tissue.

Management of Traction Detachments. The management of retinal detachment that is a consequence of proliferative diabetic retinopathy is still in a state of change. Until the advent of vitrectomy, traction detachments were often treated by encircling the globe and draining the subretinal fluid, and, in some instances, by scleral resection. When a retinal break could be identified, the preferred method of treatment was a scleral buckling procedure to seal the break. At present, combined vitrectomy and scleral buckling offers a new method of treating traction detachment, but long-term results are not yet available.

RETINAL VEIN OCCLUSION

After diabetes mellitus, the most common cause of proliferative retinopathy is probably an occlusion of one of the tributaries of the central retinal vein, which produces a classic, easily recognized ophthalmoscopic picture. In a study of the natural history of temporal branch vein occlusion, Gutman and Zegarra[27] selected 40 patients who had been periodically examined and observed for a minimum of one year. The patients ranged in age from 38 to 73 years; 33 patients (84%) were between the ages of 50 and 73 years.

Associated Vascular Problems

During the follow-up period, which ranged from 12 months to 11 years, evidence of systemic vascular disease was noted in 34 patients (85%). The etiological diagnoses included hypertension in 30 patients (75%), systemic vascular complications associated with myocardial infarction in one patient, cerebral vascular accident in one patient with diabetes mellitus, and polycythemia vera in one patient. No etiological diagnoses were made in 6 patients (15%); the results of medical studies were negative.[27]

Affected Vein

The involved vein belonged to the distribution of the superior temporal branch vein in 25 eyes of the 40 patients (63%). The increased incidence of occlusion in this area correlates with the larger number of arteriovenous crossings present in this location as compared to other areas of the retina. In 15 eyes of the 40 patients (38%), the obstruction involved the inferior temporal branch vein or its tributaries.[27]

Complications of Vein Occlusion

The two most significant complications of temporal retinal branch vein occlusions which lead to reduced visual acuity are macular edema and neovascularization of the retina. In the 40 patients evaluated by Gutman and Zagarra, the most frequently observed complication was macular edema, which was noted in 23 eyes (58%) at some time during the course of follow-up. Other macular sequelae included a macular hole, surface wrinkling retinopathy, serous retinal detachment, microaneurysmal changes in the macula, granularity of the retinal pigment epithelium hemorrhage, and macular exudates (Fig. 6-7).

Intraretinal neovascularization and microaneurysms within the area drained by the obstructed branch retinal vein were seen in 29 eyes (73%). In nine eyes (23%), preretinal neovascularization developed and was complicated in eight patients (20%) by vitreous hemorrhage. In addition, one patient with a preretinal frond developed a shallow rhegmatogenous retinal detachment secondary to two operculated tears adjacent to an area of preretinal neovascularization.

Archer, Ernest, and Newell, in a study of 95 patients with branch vein occlusion, classified their patients on the basis of adequacy of arterial perfusion, compensation of the microvasculature, and severity of retinal ischemia.[3] They noted that when retinal arterial and capillary perfusion was adequate, visual acuity was normal or near normal. If the retinal ischemia was focal, neovascularization did not develop, but if the ischemia was widespread, there was, just as in diabetes mellitus, neovascularization both locally and at the optic disc.

Ultimately, some patients with retinal vein occlusion may develop intractable vitreous hemorrhage and traction retinal detachment requiring

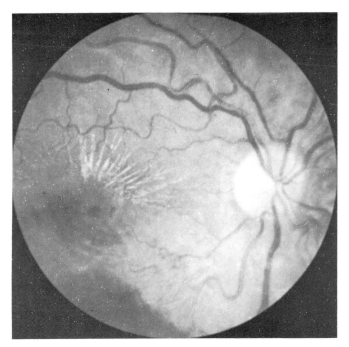

FIG. 6-7. Patient with branch vein occlusion demonstrating hemorrhage and exudation in the posterior pole.

surgical repair. Fortunately, however, many do not progress to this phase of the disease and therefore require only observation, with an attempt to establish any associated systemic etiology.

SICKLE CELL RETINOPATHY

Sickle cell disease is another cause of proliferative retinopathy. The hemoglobin of patients with sickle cell anemia (Hb S) differs from normal adult hemoglobin (Hb A). Sickling depends upon the propensity of sickle cell hemoglobin to become insoluble and gel when deoxygenated, resulting in viscous aggregates of sickled erythrocytes which may cause vascular obstruction. Other abnormal hemoglobins, identified by electrophoresis, are Hb C and Hb D. The association of sickle cell hemoglobin (Hb S) with sickle cell thalassemia (S-Thal) has also been reported. Hemoglobin S-C disease, however, is the most common variant of sickle cell disease. In 1965, Welch and Goldberg [54] examined 143 patients, 105 with abnormal hemoglobins and 38 controls. Included among the patients with abnormal hemoglobin were those with sickle cell anemia (SS), those with Hb C disease (S-C), and those with sickle cell trait (A-S). Patients with sickle cell anemia characteristically demonstrated significant venous tortuosity of the fundus and disc-shaped black retinal scars, designated the "black sunburst" sign (Fig. 6-8). Vitreous hemorrhages occurred in sickle cell anemia cases, but were rare. Patients with Hb

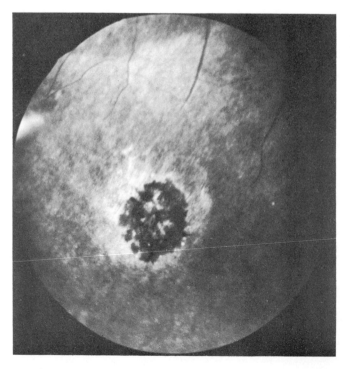

FIG. 6-8. Black sunburst sign in patient with sickle cell.

S-C disease had characteristic arteriovenous vascular fans which projected into the vitreous. This vascular abnormality was designated the "sea fan" sign because of its appearance (see Fig. 6-9). Vitreous hemorrhages were common in this group. Patients with sickle cell trait did not always have benign fundi: several patients had pathologic changes related to intravascular sickling and thrombosis.

Classification

In subsequent studies, Goldberg[24] used indirect ophthalmoscopy and fluorescein angiography to classify the sequence of fundus changes in patients with Hb S-C disease into five naturally occurring progressive stages, one leading into the next:

Stage I	Peripheral arteriolar occlusions
Stage II	Peripheral arteriolar-venular anastomoses
Stage III	Neovascular and fibrous proliferations
Stage IV	Vitreous hemorrhage
Stage V	Retinal detachment

Each of these five stages was further subdivided in order to quantify the circumferential extent of the fundus involvement:

Substage 0	No circumferential involvement
Substage 1	Circumferential involvement of up to 30 degrees of the fundus
Substage 2	Circumferential involvement of 31 to 60 degrees of the fundus
Substage 3	Circumferential involvement of 61 to 90 degrees of the fundus
Substage 4	Circumferential involvement of 91 or more degrees of the fundus

In Stage I (peripheral arteriolar occlusions), the vasculature in the posterior pole of the retina showed little or no abnormality by indirect ophthalmoscopy and fluorescein angiography in almost all cases. However, the peripheral retinal vasculature, particularly between the equator and the ora serrata, was markedly abnormal, with most of the vessels showing evidence of arteriolar obstruction. The most obvious obstructions were in the temporal quadrants. Arterioles in these locations were either totally invisible or had been converted in their terminal branches to resemble silver wires. A frequent clue to peripheral retinal ischemia was a blurred retinal appearance that obscured the underlying choroidal markings. Acute ischemic retinal edema (cloudy swelling) was not observed, possibly because of the paucity of ganglion cells, possibly because of overall thinness of the peripheral retina, or possibly because by chance the acute episodes of occlusion were not observed.

In Stage II (peripheral arteriolar-venular anastomoses) it was sometimes difficult to identify anastomoses of small peripheral arterioles or venules with indirect ophthalmoscopy. Fluorescein angiograms, however, were helpful for precise classification. As in Stage I, lesions were found in most eyes; they were frequently adjacent to Stage I lesions. Stage II was also characterized by intraluminal retention of fluorescein. No extravascular leakage of fluorescein or staining of vascular walls was observed, even when angiograms were taken 30 to 45 minutes after injection. Because fluorescein leakage characterizes most, if not all, forms of retinal neovascularization, the absence of leakage in Stage II was taken as evidence that the abnormal arterioles represent enlarged preexisting vessels, possibly capillaries, rather than newly formed vessels.

In Stage III (neovascular and fibrous proliferations) fluorescein angiography was again helpful, especially where small tufts were present; patches of neovascular and fibrous proliferations invariably leaked with the administration of intravenous fluorescein (Figs. 6-9 and 6-10). Proliferative patches apparently arise from preexisting (Stage II) arteriolar-venular anastomoses, and may possibly arise prior to the development of arteriolar-venular connections, but the angiographic evidence appeared to indicate the reverse sequence in many cases. The direction of growth of proliferative patches was generally anterior, that is, into or towards the preequatorial ischemic retina, a finding similar to that seen in diabetic retinopathy.

In Stage IV (vitreous hemorrhage) the hemorrhage usually occured sporadically without demonstrable systemic or exogenous factors. In most cases, a neovascular patch could be demonstrated as the source of the hemorrhage. The role of vitreous contraction and hemorrhage in proliferative sickle cell retinopathy (PSR) seemed less clear than in proliferative diabetic retinopathy. The hemorrhages in PSR often seemed to remain localized in the cortical vitreous which overlay the responsible patch of proliferative retinopathy. These localized vitreous hemorrhages were frequently asymptomatic, even in the presence of the usually intact peripheral visual field, and were observed only if routine ophthalmoscopy was performed at a fortuitous time. Occasionally, however, vitreous hemorrhage extended into the visual axis or into the premacular area, thereby causing visual symptoms, including reduced visual acuity.

Stage V (retinal detachment) is the ultimate and most severe stage of sickle cell retinopathy. Because such detachments were frequently related to adjacent vitreous changes, they assumed a temporal equatorial configuration similar to the configurations of the previous Stages I through IV. Retinal tears which were both round and horseshoe in shape were often found adjacent to neovascular proliferations (Fig. 6-11).

Pathogenesis

All events in sickle cell disease can be related to the sickling phenomenon, which in turn may be considered a response to ischemia and hypoxia, according to Charache and Conley.[7] A comparative study of proliferative retinopathies associated with other diseases (retrolental fibroplasia, diabetes

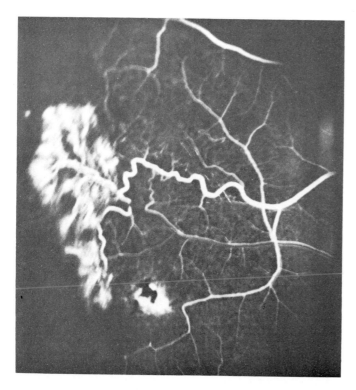

FIG. 6-9. Fluorescein angiogram of patient with hemoglobin S-C disease, showing the typical "sea fan" in the periphery.

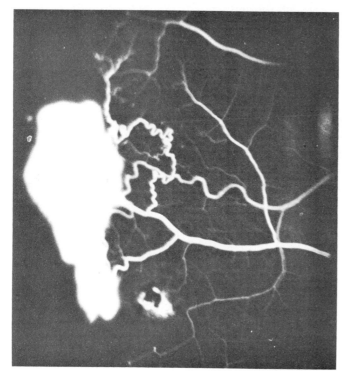

FIG. 6-10. Hemoglobin S-C disease: Late angiogram showing leakage of fluorescein dye from the sea fan.

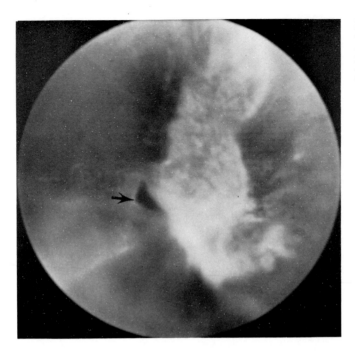

FIG. 6-11. Retinal break (the posterior margin of proliferans (*arrow*) in a patient with hemoglobin disease.

mellitus, hypertensive vascular diseases, Takayasu's [pulseless disease]) is of value in underscoring the apparent importance of ischemia in the development of proliferative sickle cell retinopathy. In retrolental fibroplasia, Patz[41] and others[44, 45] have shown that vasoconstriction and ischemia are the primary effects of hyperoxia on the immature retina. In addition, hyperoxia has a direct cytotoxic destructive effect on the neovascular endothelium, resulting in obliteration of the lumen in an affected vessel. When normal oxygen levels are restored, vasoproliferation into ischemic areas of the retina occurs as a secondary response. The peripheral and temporal predilection of this proliferative retinopathy, as well as the apparent purposeful attempt at revascularization of an ischemic retinal area, obviously resembles Stage III of proliferative sickle cell retinopathy.

In diabetes mellitus, Davis and associates[13] have suggested that ischemia is the underlying pathogenetic factor responsible for all stages of diabetic retinopathy, especially the proliferative phase. Taylor and Dobree[49] have shown that proliferative diabetic retinopathy preferentially affects the retinal quadrants in a pattern similar to that of proliferative sickle cell retinopathy, i.e., in the order superior temporal, inferior temporal, superior nasal, inferior nasal.

According to reports reviewed by Knox,[31, 32] ischemia of the retina may also be the primary factor in retinal neovascularization associated with atheromatosis or surgically induced carotid insufficiency. Fluorescein angiography has revealed that ischemia plays a similar role in the proliferative retinopathy of Takayasu's disease.

Treatment

In the treatment of proliferative sickle cell retinopathy, patches can be effectively obliterated if closure of the feeder arterioles can be accomplished as they enter the neovascular patches. Evidence suggests that argon laser photocoagulation is effective, but whether it is more effective and less dangerous than xenon arc photocoagulation of the neovascular tufts has not yet been determined.

SICKLE CELL THALASSEMIA

In another study, Goldberg, Charache, and Acacio[26] observed vascular abnormalities in the eyes of 14 patients with sickle cell thalassemia (S-Thal). Black sunbursts, seen more commonly in the fundi of patients with sickle cell anemia than in those with Hb SC disease, were seen infrequently in the fundi of patients with S-Thal. However, proliferative sickle cell retinopathy, which is much more characteristic of Hb S-C disease than of sickle cell anemia, occurred in 9 of the patients with S-Thal. The retinas of S-Thal patients thus resemble more closely those of patients with Hb S-C disease than with sickle cell anemia. The hemoglobin composition of a patient's red blood cells can be predicted to a degree from the presence and type of certain retinal abnormalities in sickling disorders, whereas the overall clinical status is not usually as good an indicator of hemoglobin composition.

In one patient, Goldberg et al.[26] noted the presence of angioid streaks in Bruch's membrane, separating the retina from the choroid. This is the first time that angioid streaks were observed in a patient with S-Thal. This finding has been reported previously in sickle cell anemia and Hb S-C diseases but rarely occurs, in our experience. The pathogenesis of the angioid streaks remains obscure in these diseases; it is possible that chronic hemolytic anemia may result in the chronic deposition of iron in Bruch's membrane, increasing its brittleness and leading to crack formation.

SARCOIDOSIS

Sarcoidosis (see also in Chap. 5) is another condition with peripheral neovascular changes. Typically this disease is associated with anterior and posterior uveitis and with sheathing of the retinal blood vessels. Sarcoid granulomas in the posterior fundus and on the optic nerve have also been observed. Less commonly recognized are the peripheral vascular changes which may arise as arteriolar-venular connections similar to those seen in the retinopathy of Hb S-C disease (Figs. 6-12 and 6-13). Thus, if they occur in a black patient, they are frequently mistaken for sickle cell disease; only after careful diagnostic workup can the correct diagnosis be established. If left unchecked, these arteriolar-venular connections may develop into neovascular tufts which ultimately cause vitreous hemorrhage and can lead to traction retinal detach-

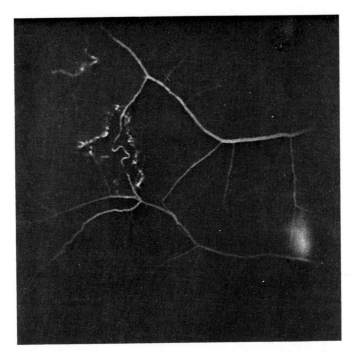

FIG. 6-12. Early arteriolar venular communication i patient with sarcoidosis.

FIG. 6-13. Arteriolar-venular connection in sarcoidosis: Late angiogram begins to show leakage from the new vessel formation.

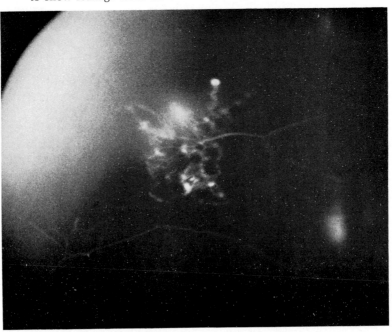

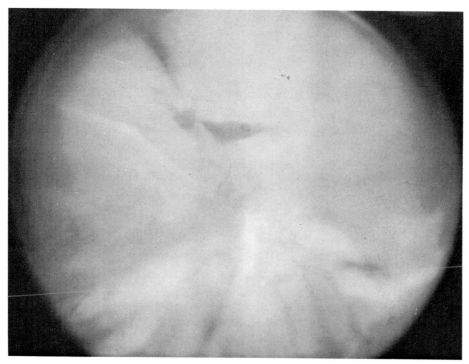

FIG. 6-14. Traction retinal detachment in a 27-year-old female with confirmed sarcoidosis.

ment (Fig. 6-14). When flat, the neovascular tufts are amenable to photocoagulation with either argon or xenon.

RETROLENTAL FIBROPLASIA

Oxygen treatment is life-saving in the neonatal respiratory distress syndrome, but unfortunately monitoring of arterial oxygen levels is difficult and retrolental fibroplasia (RLF, or retinopathy of prematurity) may develop. The solution to this clinical dilemma depends to a considerable extent on the degree of maturation of the developing retinal vasculature. At present, it is believed that upon maturation the retinal vessels are insensitive to the levels of oxygen that are attainable in arterial blood. Accordingly, the gestational age at which vascular maturation can be anticipated or clinically recognized is of the utmost importance to the pediatrician and the neonatal ophthalmologist.

Retinal Vascular Development

Studies of retinal vascular development in infants have varied in techniques, criteria of maturation, and conclusions. Histologic studies by Mann indicated that the retinal vessels emerge from the optic disc at about the 4th month of gestation and reach the ora serrata by the 8th month.[37] A subsequent study by Cogan of trypsin-digested retinas demonstrated that vascular remodeling was not complete until the 2nd or 3rd month after birth.[10] However, Fletcher concluded that the retinal vessels were usually mature at a fetal weight of 2000 grams (between the 8th and 9th month).[19] Using ink injection of the developing vessels in enucleated eyes, Michaelson found earlier and more extensive development of vessels temporally than nasally.[38] He and all other investigators, however, recognize that during the later stages of retinal vessel development the region of nonvascularized peripheral retina is always greater temporally. Foos and Kopelow, studying the retinal vasculature in eyes from infants at autopsy, described vascular maturation in 10 percent of infants at 7 gestational months.[23]

Pathogenetic Mechanisms

The early phases of retrolental fibroplasia are characterized primarily by retinal ischemia, which is produced by a vaso-occlusive effect of excessive oxygen on the immature retinal vasculature. In newborn premature infants the temporal vasculature is more immature than that of other areas, so that the major effects of hyperoxygenation begin temporally. This anatomical pre-dilection for the temporal portions of the retina is similar to that observed in other proliferative retinopathies such as diabetic and sickle cell retinopathy.

The precise mechanism by which oxygen induces vaso-obliteration of the immature retinal capillaries is unknown, but may include a direct effect on the immature capillary endothelium, pressure on the capillary caused by fluid in surrounding retinal tissue, and possibly other factors. Following a return to normal environmental oxygen levels, the premature infant's peripherally ischemic retina becomes relatively hypoxic, since it no longer obtains sufficient oxygen from surrounding tissues, including the choroid. Tortuosity of the retinal vasculature appears, along with budding of the capillary endothelium and an advancing proliferation of neovascular tissue towards the ischemic retina, which lies between the equator and the ora serrata. Fortunately, up to 80 percent of the eyes show spontaneous regression of the neovascular tissue. When the neovascularization is progressive, however, local hemorrhage and fibrous proliferations may occur.

ACTIVE RETROLENTAL FIBROPLASIA

The acute active phases of retrolental fibroplasia may be observed between the 3rd and 5th weeks of life and may last for 3 to 6 months. If progression is rapid, early retinal detachment may occur. The detachment may remain localized, causing retinal folds, or may involve the entire retina; occasionally, it resolves spontaneously.

Retrolental fibroplasia can be divided into the vaso-obliterative stage, which occurs while the infant is still receiving oxygen, and the vasoproliferative stage, which occurs after the oxygen is removed. The area of vaso-occlusion determines the site at which the vasoproliferation will develop (Fig. 6-15). Ashton and Patz et al.[3a, 42] have shown that newborn kittens given oxygen can develop vaso-obliteration of the retinal vessels all the way back to the disc; when then exposed to room air, the kittens develop neovascularization at the site of the disc.

O'Grady and associates[40] demonstrated that in the vasoproliferative stage a vascular demarcation line may occur, again usually in the temporal periphery. This area represents a large arteriovenous shunt composed of proliferating capillaries and mesenchymal cells (Fig. 6-16). If new vessels do not begin to grow across this vascular demarcation line, one can expect the development of a more severe form of retrolental fibroplasia. If, however, within the first 6 to 8 weeks new vessels develop anterior to the grey line, regression of the retrolental fibroplasia is more likely.

Classification of Active Retrolental Fibroplasia

McCormick[34] and Kingham[30] have suggested new classifications of active retrolental fibroplasia which are much more in keeping with the changes just discussed than the original classification, and are more helpful to the ophthalmologist. Basically McCormick describes four stages. Stage I is that of early neovascularization. In Stage II, neovascularization begins to enter the vitreous cavity. By Stage III affected infants start to show dilatation and increased tortuosity of the retinal vessels in the posterior pole, and finally, in Stage IV, some degree of retinal detachment is noted. This active phase may continue for up to 6 months after birth or may terminate sooner. As a result it is

FIG. 6-15. Retrolental fibroplasia: Diagram showing spasm of peripheral vessels on the temporal side followed by early neovascularization in the area of anoxia.

ACTIVE RLF

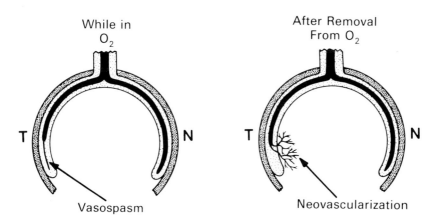

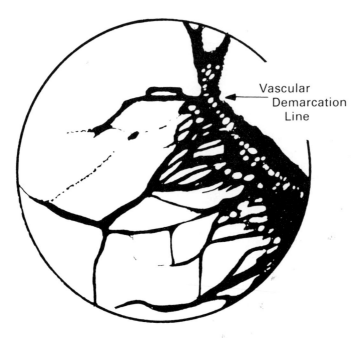

Vascular
Demarcation
Line

FIG. 6-16. Vascular
demarcation line in act
retrolental fibroplasia (I
Growth of vessels anter
the demarcation line
suggests regression of t
RLF.

sometimes difficult to recognize precisely when the active phase has ended
and the cicatricial phase has begun.

CICATRICIAL RETROLENTAL FIBROPLASIA

Findings in cicatricial retrolental fibroplasia may also be divided into differ-
ing grades of severity on the basis of fundus changes:

Grade I	Myopia
	Peripheral retinal pigmentation
	Frosting on peripheral retina
	Peripheral vitreous membranes
	Equatorial retinal folds
Grade II	Grade I plus
	Dragging of the retina in the posterior pole
	Neovascularization
	Elevated retinal vessels
	Retinal breaks
Grade III	Falciform retinal folds
Grade IV	Rhegmatogenous retinal detachment
	Exudative retinal detachment
Grade V	Organized retinal detachment

All gradations from very slight damage to total organized retinal detachment
may be found, regardless of the infant's birth weight or gestational age. Thus,

a child weighing less than 1 kilogram (2.2 lb.) at birth may exhibit only myopia, whereas a patient weighing close to 2.25 kilograms (5 lb.) at birth may develop organized retinal detachment.

Grade I

Myopia. One of the most common findings associated with retrolental fibroplasia is myopia. In our experience it occurs in over 80 percent of children with cicatricial retrolental fibroplasia, and is usually more than 6 diopters.[46] It occurs early and falls into the congenital group of myopias as defined by Hiatt et al.[28] It may be noted within the first 2 months of life and may progress during the first 6 years. Although the cause of the myopia is obscure, there appears to be a significant relationship between the degree of myopia and the severity of retrolental fibroplasia. Fletcher and Brandon noted that premature infants who developed retrolental fibroplasia retained their early myopia, whereas those who did not develop retrolental fibroplasia lost their myopia by the age of one year.[20] This relationship is important, since retinal detachment, a severe consequence of cicatricial retrolental fibroplasia, occurs most often in highly myopic eyes.

Whether or not myopia in retrolental fibroplasia is axial or is due to other abnormalities, such as corneal or lenticular changes or shallowing of the anterior chamber, remains in question. The axial lengths of ten retrolental fibroplasia patients varying in age from 3 months to 21 years were measured with the aid of A-scan ultrasound. These lengths were then correlated with refractive errors. Some of the axial lengths were within the range of normal for an emmetrope of the same age despite the fact that the patients were myopic. On the other hand, nine of the patients had myopia more marked in one eye than the other, and in six of these patients a longer axial length was present in the more myopic eye, suggesting that multiple factors may be responsible, one of which is elongation of the eye.

Retinal Pigmentation. Alterations in the pigmentation of the fundus are common in cicatricial retrolental fibroplasia and may be found in the posterior pole as well as the fundus periphery. Pigment clumping similar to that seen in hyperplasia of the pigment epithelium (see in Chap. 7) may occur, as well as discrete patches characterized by loss of the pigment epithelium and outer sensory retinal layers.

Vitreous Membranes. In mild cicatricial retrolental fibroplasia, peripheral vitreous membranes develop anterior to the equator, especially on the temporal side (Fig. 6-17). These may be present when there are no alterations in the posterior pole. However, the converse is not true. If posterior pole changes, such as dragging of the retina, are detected, peripheral changes will almost invariably be present.

In neonates the presence of peripheral vitreous membranes has a much more ominous significance than it has in older patients, since many such neonates are still in the resolving active phase. During this period of time, they may show a limited temporal retinal detachment. Quite often such

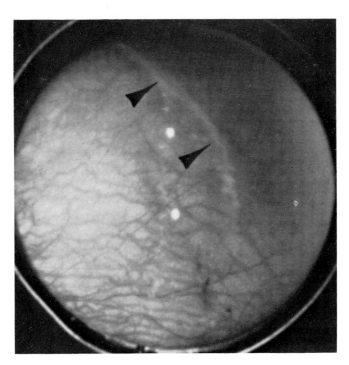

FIG. 6-17. Cicatricial retrolental fibroplasia: Peripheral vitreous membranes (*arrows*) temporally in a 3-month-old infant.

detachments have a tractional component, but since they may resolve spontaneously, exudation secondary to traction on the retinal vessels also appears to be a factor. Demarcation lines sometimes delimit the posterior margin of the detachment and in later life may be the only residual clue that retinal elevation once existed.

Equatorial Retinal Folds. Equatorial retinal folds usually occur between the equator and the ora serrata and may be the sole retinal findings consistent with ciacatricial retolental fibroplasia. They are found at the location of the vascular demarcation line (described by O'Grady, Flynn, and Jerrera[40]) which was present during the active phase of retrolental fibroplasia, and are often associated with areas of retinal pigmentation. The retinal vessels cross the folds and travel anteriorly towards the ora serrata.

Grade II

Dragging of the Retina. Displaced (dragged) retinas are a hallmark of cicatricial retrolental fibroplasia (Fig. 6-18).[46, 18] In 80 percent of the cases, dragging or displacement is to the temporal side, and frequently the macula may be displaced temporally as well, causing pseudoheterotropia. Pigmentary changes in the macular area are also common. It is usual for the dragging of the disc and macula to be significantly greater in one eye than in the other, since asymmetry is a characteristic of retrolental fibroplasia (Figs. 6-19 and 6-20). One eye may even approach phthisis while the other retains good visual function and appears nearly normal.

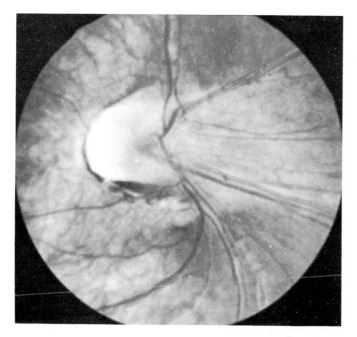

FIG. 6-18. Cicatricial retrolental fibroplasia: Typical dragging of the retina to the temporal side.

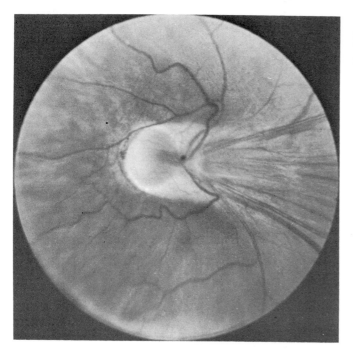

FIG. 6-19. Cicatricial retrolental fibroplasia: Temporal dragging of the retina.

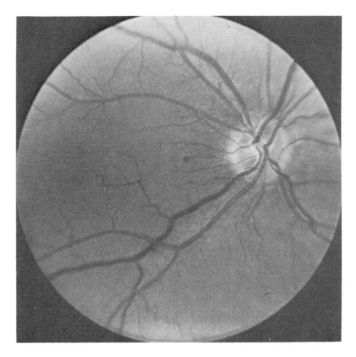

FIG. 6-20. Fellow eye of patient shown in Figure [illegible] The disc is normal, illustrating the asymmetr[y] which frequently occurs [in] retrolental fibroplasia.

The histologic examination of eyes with dragged retinas reveals several interesting observations. Importantly, the retina is folded over the optic nerve, while the nerve itself may show little or no displacement. Therefore, the term dragged retina has been suggested, to replace dragged disc.

Neovascularization. A less common peripheral retinal finding is neovascularization of the retina (Fig. 6-21) which, as in other proliferative retinopathies, occurs in close proximity to areas of retinal ischemia.

These areas, frequently difficult to detect, may give rise to vitreous hemorrhage during the teenage or early adult years. Fluorescein angiography and angioscopy are helpful aids in documenting neovascular sites, which, if symptomatic in teenagers or young adults, are best treated by laser or cryotherapy.

Elevated Retinal Vessels. Elevated retinal vessels may be seen in patients with cicatricial retrolental fibroplasia.[46] The elevated vessels leave the retina and run along the posterior surface of the focally detached vitreous gel.

As in the case of neovascularization, elevated vessels can give rise to vitreous hemorrhage. Their management, however, is much more difficult because they are large in caliber and difficult to obliterate by any means. Generally, the hemorrhages clear spontaneously and visual acuity returns to the prehemorrhagic level. Therefore, no treatment at all is the best treatment, but patients with this problem should be advised to refrain from contact sports and other jarring activities.

Lattice Degeneration. Lattice degeneration in patients with cicatricial retrolental fibroplasia is similar to that seen in patients who have no history of prematurity (see Lattice Degeneration in Chap. 8). Generally, there is a thinning of the inner retinal layers, coupled with a vitreous condensation over the area of lattice degeneration. These areas frequently develop retinal break formation. (Fig. 6-22).

Lattice degeneration was noted in 13 out of 85 patients (15%) with cicatricial retrolental fibroplasia. This is considerably higher than the 6 to 7 percent incidence reported in the general population. Because of the associated high myopia and increased incidence of retinal detachment in these patients, cryotherapy, applied to areas of retinal break formation within the lattice, is recommended.

Retinal Breaks. Retinal breaks which occur in cicatricial retrolental fibroplasia tend to be located primarily on the temporal side. Usually, they are round or oval in shape and equatorial in location. As just mentioned, they may occur in association with lattice degeneration. Marked equatorial folds indicative of severe vitreous traction are common just anterior to the breaks. Operculated tears have also been noted, as well as breaks close to the optic nerve, and giant retinal tears. All breaks should be treated prophylactically. An encircling scleral buckling procedure is indicated because of the importance and the progressive nature of the vitreoretinal traction in cicatricial retrolental fibroplasia. Follow-up examinations of the ocular fundi are done every 6 months, with emphasis on peripheral retinal examination to look for new retinal breaks.

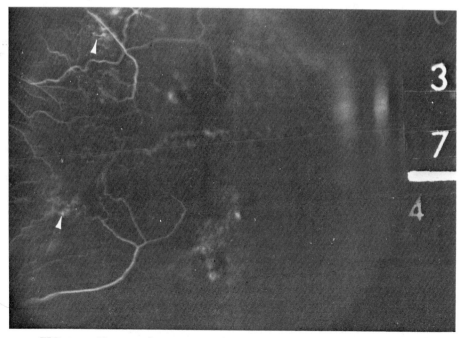

FIG. 6-21. Neovascularization (*arrows*) in a teenager with mild cicatricial retrolental fibroplasia.

Grade III—Falciform Retinal Fold

In more severe cases of cicatricial retrolental fibroplasia, dragging of the retina assumes the shape of a retinal fold, again most commonly located on the temporal side. Usually the fold runs through the macula towards the fundus periphery.

The cortical vitreous is thickened over the fold and is adherent to it. Retinal vessels which are incorporated into the retinal fold give the surrounding fundus a relatively avascular appearance. In the periphery the retinal fold fans out to terminate in a gliotic mass at the vitreous base. Despite all of these changes, however, retinal detachment is rare in eyes with falciform retinal folds.

Because retinal folds frequently run through the macular area, ocular nystagmus and amblyopia are associated findings. To minimize the nystagmus and improve visual acuity, affected youngsters will often turn their heads slightly to abduct the better eye. It is not uncommon for folds to occur in one eye while the other eye appears relatively normal, suggesting that many of the congenital retinal folds first described by Mann[37] may actually be forms of asymmetrical cicatricial retrolental fibroplasia, even in full-term infants.

Grade IV—Retinal Detachment

One of the most serious complications of cicatricial retrolental fibroplasia is retinal detachment. We have now operated on 55 such detachments in 50

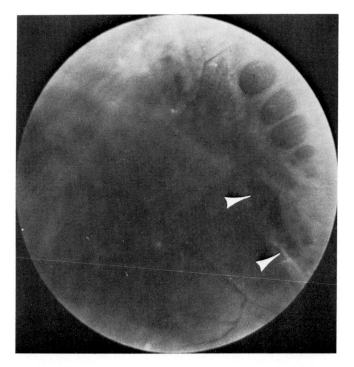

FIG. 6-22. Cicatricial retrolental fibroplasia: Lattice (*arrows*) with retina holes.

patients ranging in age from 5 weeks to 27 years. Of these detachments, 39 were rhegmatogenous and 16 were tractional exudative detachments.

In the rhegmatogenous detachments multiple rather than single retinal breaks are the rule, and the incidence of detachment is greater in children whose birth weight was under 1500 grams than in those who had a higher birth weight. The most common age at onset is 14 years, but rhegmatogenous detachments also occur in patients under ten and over twenty. Retinal breaks and their treatments are discussed above.

Tractional exudative retinal detachment occurs in both infants and young adults, but the average age, 5.7 years, is much lower than for patients with rhegmatogenous retinal detachment. Exudation in all age groups is related to vitreous traction on temporal peripheral vessels. Our treatment consisted of a scleral buckling procedure utilizing cryotherapy to eliminate the abnormal vasculature. In infants a no. 40 silicone band was used, and the ends were either abutted or left long so that the tension on the globe could be released later if intrusion became a problem owing to growth of the eye. It is important to remember that an infant's eye is considerably smaller than an adult's and may have an axial length as short as 15 mm. Children over 1 year old were treated with silicone rubber buckling beneath scleral flaps and a no. 40 band. Of seven eyes treated with an encircling buckle alone, all but one showed retinal reattachment, although one patient treated successfully required two procedures. Despite reattachment, however, three eyes did not regain visual function and continued to demonstrate a flat electroretinogram.

Vitrectomy has also been attempted in retrolental fibroplasia.[51] In our experience the results have been disappointing, quite possibly owing to failure to remove the cortical vitreous from the retinal surface, since vitreous detachment is rare in these patients. Finally, of special importance is the fact that temporal peripheral retinal detachments in infants occasionally resolve spontaneously.

On the basis of our experience with these cases, we have come to recognize that increased tortuosity of the retinal vessels in the posterior pole in infants and accumulation of subretinal exudation (Fig. 6-23) are ominous signs invariably followed by a downhill course. For this reason, if these changes are noted early we now feel that surgical intervention is indicated, using scleral buckling, vitrectomy, and sometimes a combination of both modalities. For newborns without exudation, it has been our policy to withhold surgery unless the detachment extends into the macula, since, as noted above, peripheral detachments may flatten without treatment.

Grade V—Organized Retinal Detachment

Organized retinal detachment occurs as the end stage of both acute and cicatricial retrolental fibroplasia. It may develop within the first 2 months of postnatal life and, in our experience, does not respond to any form of surgical intervention. This stage is characterized by leukocoria.

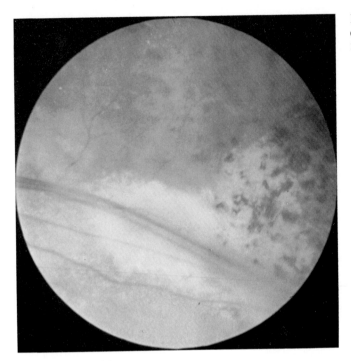

FIG. 6-23. Subretinal exudation in retrolental fibroplasia.

EALES' DISEASE

Eales' disease, characterized by recurring hemorrhages into the retina and vitreous, occurs predominantly in young males (under the age of 40) who are apparently healthy.[48] The disease starts more frequently in the left eye, but may begin in the right eye as well. Associated findings are epistaxis, constipation, and headache. Periphlebitis develops in the retinal periphery and may lead to central retinal vein obstruction. The periphlebitis may resolve spontaneously or may progress to the formation of new vessels in the areas of venous blockage. If blockage is extensive, neovascular formation may also arise on the optic nerve head. The neovascular areas can lead to massive vitreous hemorrhages which in turn may lead to proliferative retinopathy and detachment of the retina (Fig. 6-24).

Results of fluorescein angiography are suggestive of venous occlusive disease because there is leakage from retinal veins and capillaries, and profuse leakage from new vessel formations.

Etiology and Incidence

Although the etiology of Eales' disease is still obscure, the old concept is that it represents an allergic reaction of tissue previously sensitized to tuberculin protein. Eales' disease appears to be endemic in certain areas. It is much more prevalent in Western Europe and India than in the United States. In the middle Atlantic states, very few cases of Eales' disease are seen.

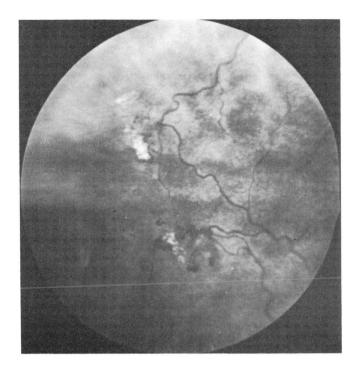

FIG. 6-24. Neovascularization in the periphery of a patient with Eales' disease.

Management

Eales' disease often undergoes spontaneous remission, making treatment unnecessary. In those cases that progress to neovascularization, photocoagulation has proved to be the treatment of choice. Neovascular fronds may be treated with either argon laser therapy or xenon photocoagulation. If neovascularization is flat on the retina, xenon photocoagulation seems preferable. If neovascularization involves the disc, argon laser therapy is the treatment of choice, particularly if the vessels on the disc have led to vitreous hemorrhage. In most patients in whom vitreous hemorrhage has not occurred from the disc vessels, only the peripheral neovascularization is treated.

Patients who either bleed initially and fail to clear or have recurrent vitreous hemorrhage following treatment may be candidates for surgical intervention, namely, pars plana vitrectomy.[30]

COATS' DISEASE (RETINAL TELANGIECTASIA)

Coats' disease, or retinal telangiectasia (perhaps a better term), is characterized by retinal vascular changes and exudation.[45] As a rule, males are predominantly affected, although Coats' disease has occurred in both sexes. Involvement is usually unilateral but bilateral cases have occurred.

Originally the disease was classified into three types: Type I, exudation present; Type II, exudation and vascular changes present; and Type III, angiomatosis retinae present.[8, 9] It is now recognized that the exudation is secondary to the vascular changes, which are frequently located in the retinal periphery. At present Coats' disease is no longer divided into types, but is divided into patient groups according to the age of the patient, one group consisting of juvenile males primarily, and the other of adults. In the adult form there is usually an associated elevated serum cholesterol, which is not present in boys, and which may be secondary to vascular occlusion or uveitis. In juvenile males, the disease may occur in infancy, but diagnosis is usually made at about 10 years of age.

Leber[33] described a condition which at one time was considered a separate entity from Coats' disease, but little distinction is made between the two conditions today. The relationship between the adult form of Coats' disease and peripheral exudative hemorrhagic chorioretinopathy is discussed under the latter condition in Chapter 8.

Retinal Findings

The classic lesion is the so-called light bulb telangiectatic change in the retinal periphery (Plate 1, *A* and *B*). The vascular changes are most common in the superior temporal quadrant, but may involve any quadrant. Ultimately, the lesions lead to a yellow subretinal exudation which is found in the periphery and the posterior pole (Fig. 6-25).

With fluorescein angiography, the telangiectatic "light bulb" can leak fluorescein profusely, in contrast to a cavernous retinal hemangioma (see in Chap. 7), in which the fluorescein gravitates within the lesion and is retained for a long period of time (Figs. 6-26 and 6-27). The larger vessels within an affected area often show dilatation and beading of the wall as well as aneurysmal formation and total or partial vein occlusion. The arteriovenous channels become prominent and loss of the capillary bed can be observed (Fig. 6-28).

Changes in the larger vessels are more pronounced close to an area of diseased retina. The smaller retinal vascular changes, in which loss of the normal capillary bed occurs, are accompanied by large arteriovenous communications. On fluorescein angiography microaneurysmal changes are also apparent; these are most commonly found in areas of diffuse capillary loss.

Differential Diagnosis

The differentiation of retinal telangiectasia from retinoblastoma is discussed in Chapter 7. Retinal telangiectasia must also be differentiated from familial exudative vitreoretinopathy, a bilateral ocular disease inherited as an autosomal dominant trait. This disorder has no apparent systemic manifestations and involves primarily the vitreous body and retina. Slowly progressive vitreous contraction occurs and may lead to vitreous hemorrhage and retinal detachment. Liquefaction of the vitreous gel, however, is infrequent. Posterior pole changes include dragging of the retina that is similar to the

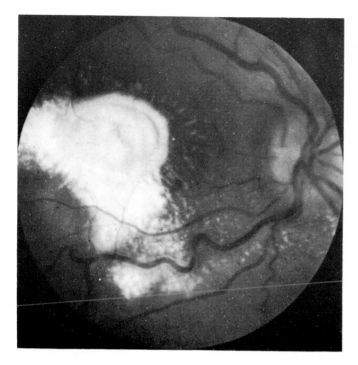

FIG. 6-25. Exudation in the macula of a patient with retinal telangiectasia.

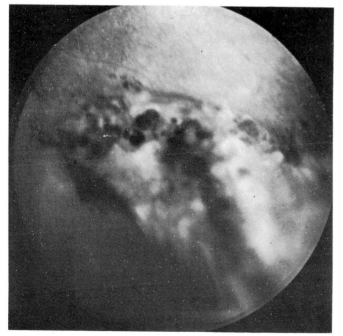

FIG. 6-26. Cavernous retinal hemangioma with gliotic tissue.

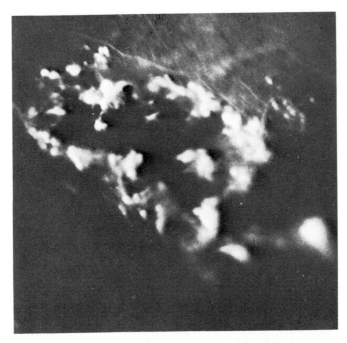

FIG. 6-27. Fluorescein within the cavernous retinal hemangioma gravitates within the saccular aneurysmal changes.

FIG. 6-28. Retinal telangiectasia showing areas of retinal ischemia. The aneurysmal changes in the posterior pole are oriented towards the anoxic zones.

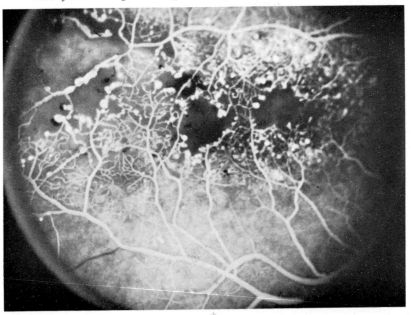

dragging seen in cicatricial retrolental fibroplasia, and displacement of the macula. Ultimately, subretinal exudation, total retinal detachment, and optic atrophy may occur.

Treatment

When the disease is found to be progressive and subretinal exudation is increasing, the goal of treatment is obliteration of the abnormal telangiectatic vascular changes. Photocoagulation or cryotherapy may be indicated. Treatment in children usually has to be carried out under general anesthesia; at that time, xenon arc photocoagulation is preferable to argon laser therapy because the patients are recumbent. However, if large amounts of exudation are present beneath the telangiectatic area, it is difficult to obtain an adequate photocoagulation reaction, and cryotherapy becomes the treatment of choice.

Prognosis and Follow-Up

The prognosis with treatment is best when only one or two quadrants are affected; prognosis worsens significantly when the disease involves more than 180 degrees of the retinal periphery. Retinal detachment may be treated by a scleral buckling procedure, at which time the vascular abnormality may be eliminated either by diathermy in a scleral bed or by cryotherapy. Subretinal fluid must be drained, and the retina may then become reattached. If all vascular abnormalities are not eliminated, subsequent laser or xenon photocoagulation on the buckle may be necessary.

In the management of Coats' disease, it is important to monitor the patient until all vascular abnormalities have been eliminated; this may require 10 to 12 months. Exudation will begin to resorb in about 6 to 8 weeks. New vascular abnormalities may develop and must be treated. Recurrence has occurred as late as 5 years after an apparent cure, so 6-month periodic check-ups are suggested.

LEUKEMIA

Leukemia rarely causes a diagnostic ocular problem since systemic involvement is usually already present. Allen and Straatsma[1] and Mahneke and Videbok[36] have emphasized the high incidence of retinal lesions in patients with leukemia. They frequently observed dilated tortuous veins, leukemic infiltrates, hemorrhages, and exudates. Hemorrhages with white centers (Roth spots) were common and sometimes extended from the inner plexiform layer to the internal limiting membrane. (Wong and Bodey[55] noted Roth spots in a patient with aplastic anemia and found that the central core contained an eosinophilic material which, when stained, had an appearance consistent with fibrin. Papilledema and retinal edema were less common findings.)

Duke, Wilkinson, and Sigelman[16] found significant numbers of retinal microaneurysms in seven of nine patients with chronic myeloid leukemia and in three of ten patients with chronic lymphoid leukemia. Generally, the aneurysms were located in the retinal periphery, a fact that might lead to their being overlooked on a casual fundus examination.

Toussaint and Farmir[50] described retinal microaneurysms in two patients with leukemia and related the occurrence of these lesions to steroid therapy. They also described peripheral microaneurysms in the retinas of 20 to 30 percent of a group of control patients, but did not cite the number of lesions per retina.

REFERENCES

1. **Allen RA, Straatsma BR:** Ocular involvement in leukemia and allied disorders. Arch Ophthalmol (66: 490–508), 1971
2. American Diabetes Association, 1978
3. **Archer DB, Ernest JR, Newell FW:** Classification of branch retina vein occlusion. Trans Amer Acad Ophthalmol Otolaryngol 78:148–165, 1974
3a. **Ashton N:** Animal experiment. Trans Amer Acad Ophthalmol 58:51, 1954
4. **Betts EK, Downes JJ, Schaffer DB, Johns R:** Retrolental fibroplasia and oxygen administration during general anesthesia. Anesthesiology 47:518–520, 1977
5. **Brockhurts R, Chishti MI:** Cicatricial retrolental fibroplasia: its occurrence without oxygen administrations and in full term infants. Albrecht von Graefes Arch Klin Ophthalmol 195:113-128, 1975
6. **Burdett AF, Caird FI, Draper GJ:** The natural history of diabetic retinopathy. Q J Med 37:303–317, 1968
7. **Charache S, Conley CL:** Rate of sickling of red cells during deoxygenation of blood from persons with various sickling disorders. Blood 24:25–48, 1964
8. **Coats G:** Forms of retinal disease with massive exudation. R Lond Ophthalmol Hosp Rep 17:440, 1908
9. **Coats G:** Ueber retinitis exudativa (retinitis hemorrhagia externa). Albrecht von Graefes Arch Klin Ophthalmol 81:275, 1912
10. **Cogan DG:** Development of senescence of the human vasculature. Doyne Memorial Lecture, 1963. Trans Ophthalmol Soc 83:465–489, 1963
11. **Cohen AM:** Lessons from diabetes in Yemenites. Isr J Med Sci 7:1554–1557, 1971
12. **Cullen JF:** Diabetic retinopathy: hope or despair. Trans Ophthalmol Soc UK 92:59–68, 1972
13. **Davis MD, et al:** Clinical observations concerning pathogenesis of diabetic retinopathy. In Goldberg MD. Fine SL (eds): Symposium on the Treatment of Diabetic Retinopathy. Washington DC, US PHS Publication No. 1890, 1969
14. Diabetic Retinopathy Study Research Group: Photocoagulation treatment of proliferative diabetic retinopathy: the second report of diabetic retinopathy findings. Trans Am Acad Ophthalmol Otolaryngol 85:82–106, 1978
15. **Dobree JH:** Proliferative diabetic retinopathy. Evolution of the retinal lesions. Br J Ophthalmol 48:637–649, 1964
16. **Duke JR, Wilkinson CP, Sigelman S:** Retinal microaneurysms in leukemia. Br J Ophthalmol 52:368–374, 1968
17. **Eastman NJ:** Williams obstetrics, 10th ed. New York, Appleton-Century-Crofts, 1950
18. **Faris B, Tolentino FI, Freeman H MacK, Brockhurst RJ, Schepens CL:** Retrolental fibroplasia in the cicatricial stage. Arch Ophthalmol 85:661–668, 1971
19. **Fletcher MC:** Retrolental fibroplasia, role of oxygen. In Report of the 16th Ross (M&R) Pediatric Research Conference. Columbus, M&R Laboratories, 1955, pp. 34–38
20. **Fletcher MC, Brandon S:** Myopia of prematurity. Am J Ophthalmol 40:474–481, 1955
21. **Flynn J:** Personal communication
22. **Flynn J, Patz A:** Personal communication
23. **Foos RY, Kopelow SM:** Development of retinal vasculature in paranatal infants. Surv Ophthalmol 18:117–127, 1973

24. **Goldberg MF:** Classification and pathogenesis of proliferative sickle retinopathy. Am J Ophthalmol 71(3):649–665, 1971

25. **Goldberg MF:** Retinal detachment associated with proliferative retinopathies (sickle cell disease, retrolental fibroplasia, and diabetes mellitus). Isr J Med Sci 8:1447–1457, 1972

26. **Goldberg MF, Charache S, Acacio I:** Ophthalmic manifestations of sickle cell thalassemia. Arch Intern Med 128:33–39, 1971

27. **Gutman FA, Zegarra H:** The natural course of temporal retinal branch vein occlusion. Trans Am Ophthalmol Soc 78:OP-178–192, 1974

28. **Hiatt RL, Costenbader FD, Albert DG:** Clinical evaluation of congenital myopia. Arch Ophthalmol 74:31–35, 1965

29. **Kahn A, Bradley RF:** Prevalence of diabetic retinopathy. Br J Ophthalmol 59:345–349, 1975

30. **Kingham J:** Acute retrolental fibroplasia. Arch Ophthalmol 95:39–47, 1977

31. **Knox DL:** Ischemic ocular inflammation. Am J Ophthalmol 60:995–1002, 1965

32. **Knox DL:** Ocular aspects of cervical vascular disease. Surv Ophthalmol 13:245–262, 1969

33. **Leber TH:** Retinitis exudativa (Coats), retinitis und chorioretinitis serofibrinosa degenerans. Albrecht von Graefes Arch Klin Ophthalmol 7:1267, 1915

34. **McCormick A:** The retinopathy of prematurity in the newborn. Curr Prob Pediatr 7:3028, 1977

35. **McMeel JW:** Diabetic retinopathy: fibrotic proliferation and retinal detachment.Trans Am Ophthalmol Soc 69:440–493, 1971

36. **Mahneke A, Videbok A:** On changes in the optic fundus in leukemia. Arch Ophthalmol 42:201–210, 1964

37. **Mann I:** The Development of the Human Eye, 3rd ed. New York, Grune & Stratton, 1964

38. **Michaelson IC:** Retinal Circulation in Man and Animals. 1954, pp 95–100 CC Thomas, Springfield, IL

39. **Oakley N, Hill DW, Joplin FG, Kohner E, Fraser TR:.**Diabetic retinopathy. Diabetologia 3:402–405, 1967

40. **O'Grady GE, Flynn JT Jerrera JA:** The clinical course of retrolental fibroplasia in premature infants. South Med J 65:655–658, 1972

41. **Patz A:** The continuing role of the ophthalmologist in the premature nursery. Arch Ophthalmol 85:129–130, 1971

42. **Patz A, Eastham A, Higginbotham DH, Kleh T:** Oxygen studies in retrolental fibroplasia. II. The production of the microscopic changes of retrolental fibroplasia in experimental animals. Am J Ophthalmol 36:1511–1522, 1953

43. **Silverman WA:** Durham's Premature Infants. New York, Hoeber, 1961

44. **Tasman W:** Vitreoretinal changes in cicatricial retrolental fibroplasia. Trans Am Ophthalmol Soc 68:548–594, 1970

45. **Tasman W:** Coat's disease. In Tasman W (ed): Retinal Diseases in Children. New York, Harper & Row, 1971, pp 59–69

46. **Tasman W:** Retrolental fibroplasia. In Tasman W (ed): Retinal Diseases in Children. New York, Harper & Row, 1971, pp 105–120

47. **Tasman W:** Retinal detachment secondary to proliferative diabetic retinopathy. Mod. Probl Ophthalmol 10:319–324, 1972

48. **Tasman W:** The present diagnostic and therapeutic approach to Eales' disease, Coats' disease, and Lebers miliary aneurysms. In: L'Esperance F (ed): Current Diagnosis and Management of Chorioretinal Disease. St. Louis, Mosby, 1977, pp 159–163

49. **Taylor E, Dobree HJ:** Proliferative diabetic retinopathy, site and size of initial lesions. Br J Ophthalmol 54:11–18, 1970

50. **Toussaint D, Farmir A:** Etude de la vascularisation retinienne de sujects traités a la cortisone. Bull Soc Belge Ophtalmol 143:568–577, 1968

51. **Treister G, Machemer R:** Results of vitrectomy for rare proliferative and hemorrhagic disease. Am J Ophthalmol 84:394–412, 1977

52. United States Department of Health, Education and Welfare, Vital Statistics of the United States. Natality 1:1, 1966

53. **Wagner HP, Wilder RM:** The retinitis of diabetic mellitus. JAMA 76:515–517, 1921

54. **Welch RB, Goldberg MF:** Sickle-cell hemoglobin and its relation to fundus abnormality. Arch Ophthalmol 75:353–362, 1966

55. **Wong V, Bodey GP:** Hemorrhagic retinoschisis due to aplastic anemia. Arch Ophthalmol 80:433–434, 1968

7

Tumors

Tumors which occur in the peripheral fundus are histologically identical to those which occur in the posterior fundus. Because of their peripheral location, however, their clinical presentation, clinical course, diagnosis, and management are often quite different from tumors of the posterior pole. This chapter will discuss tumors of the peripheral fundus and will emphasize these differences. It will consider tumors of the retina, the nonpigmented ciliary epithelium, the pigmented epithelium, and the uveal tract.

TUMORS OF THE RETINA

RETINOBLASTOMA

Retinoblastoma is the most common intraocular malignancy of childhood, occurring in about 1:18,000 live births.[7] Although recognized to be congenital, it usually becomes clinically apparent during the first or second year of life. There is no predilection for race or sex.

The etiology of retinoblastoma is not clearly understood.[4, 8] About 6 percent of patients have a positive family history, in which case the tumor is transmitted by an autosomal dominant mode of inheritance with incomplete penetrance. The other 94 percent of retinoblastomas are sporadic mutations with a negative family history. Of the sporadic cases, about 25 percent represent germinal mutations: patients have the propensity to pass the gene to their offspring. The remaining 75 percent are somatic mutations with no tendency to pass the gene on. There are possibly environmental and viral factors which play a role in the pathogenesis, but at the present time they are poorly understood.

Clinical Features

The tumor is diagnosed at an average age of 18 months, with the bilateral cases being recognized earlier. In rare cases it may be diagnosed later in life.[33] Patients with retinoblastoma usually present with leukocoria, a white pupillary reflex due to a large intraocular mass. Less commonly, the initial sign is strabismus, intraocular inflammation, vitreous hemorrhage, or glaucoma.

In many instances the retinoblastoma arises from the peripheral retina. In such cases, the tumor often attains a large size before strabismus or leukocoria occur. Small peripheral retinoblastomas are often asymptomatic and are discovered in either of two ways: (1) they may be recognized when the second eye is examined under anesthesia after discovery of a large tumor in the first eye, or (2) they may be diagnosed on routine examination of a sibling or an offspring of a patient known to have a retinoblastoma.

A peripheral retinoblastoma, which may be unifocal or multifocal, appears clinically as a small white elevated lesion located anywhere in the peripheral retina. (Plate 2, *A*). The lesion usually has a smooth surface, but it sometimes appears irregular owing to the presence of calcium within the tumor. Fairly prominent retinal vessels may supply the mass. In contrast to tumors of the posterior pole, there is usually no significant retinal detachment. Seeding of tumor cells into the vitreous is unusual with a small retinoblastoma, but may occur with larger tumors (Fig. 7-1). As the tumor becomes larger, typical leukocoria may develop. (Plate 2, *B*).

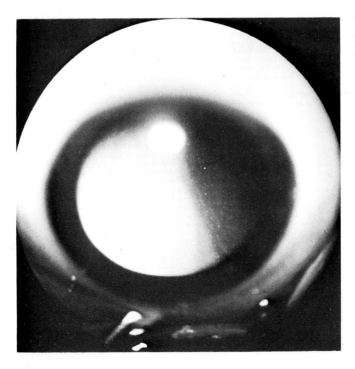

FIG. 7-1. Large peripheral endophytic retinoblastoma producing overlying vitreous seeding.

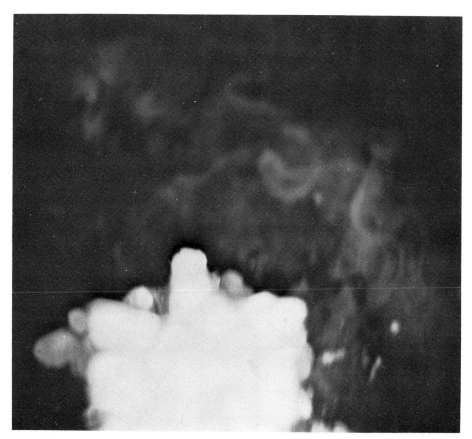

FIG. 7-2. Fundus photograph of a spontaneously regressed retinoblastoma situated near the equator inferiorly.

About 1 percent of retinoblastomas undergo spontaneous retrogression, the cause of which is unknown.[5] This appears clinically as an area of pigment dispersion and gliosis with a central mound of calcium that resembles cottage cheese (Fig. 7-2).

Pathology

Like tumors which occur in the posterior pole, peripheral retinoblastomas may assume a growth pattern that is either endophytic (Fig. 7-3) or exophytic. The tumor may arise from any of the nuclear layers of the retina. The choroid is usually uninvolved when the tumor is small, but choroidal invasion may occur with larger tumors. Cytologically, retinoblastomas range from undifferentiated to well differentiated. The undifferentiated tumor consists of poorly developed retinoblasts and areas of necrosis and calcification (Fig. 7-4). The well-differentiated tumor is characterized by Flexner-Wintersteiner rosettes (Fig. 7-5), fleurettes, and few mitotic figures.[38, 39]

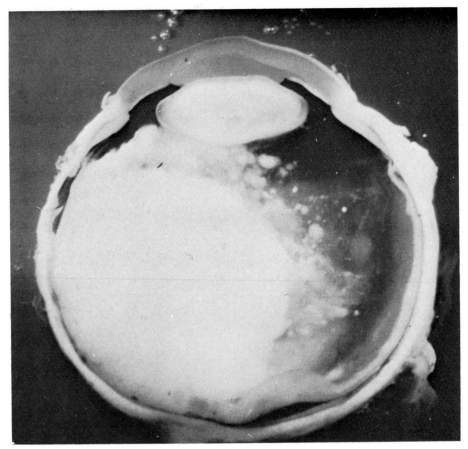

FIG. 7-3. Grossly sectioned globe showing an endophytic retinoblastoma.

Differential Diagnosis

The differential diagnosis of retinoblastoma varies with the clinical presentation of the tumor. A good deal has been written about the differential diagnosis of large tumors which produce leukocoria. Lesions such as congenital cataracts, persistent hyperplastic primary vitreous, retinopathy of prematurity (retrolental fibroplasia), nematode endophthalmitis (toxocariasis), advanced Coats' disease, and other conditions may produce a similar leukocoria.[24] Most of these disorders are discussed in other chapters. The differential diagnosis of peripheral retinoblastoma includes retinal astrocytoma, capillary hemangioma of the retina, early Coats' disease, nematode granuloma, peripheral uveoretinitis, retrolental fibroplasia, medulloepithelioma, and organized hemorrhage. Differentiation of these conditions is discussed here.

Retinal Astrocytoma. A lesion which most closely simulates a small retinoblastoma is the astrocytoma, discussed later in this chapter. Like ret-

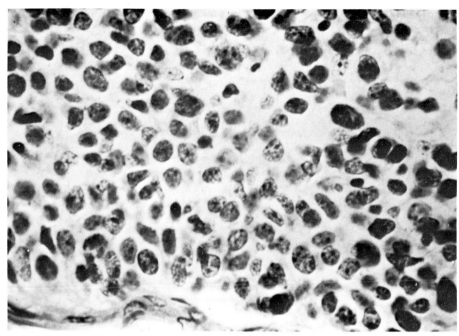

FIG. 7-4. Photomicrograph of a poorly differentiated retinoblastoma. (AFIP accession no. 1182929) (Hematoxylin-eosin stain; ×300)

FIG. 7-5. Photomicrograph of a well-differentiated retinoblastoma showing Flexner-Wintersteiner rosettes. (Hematoxylin-eosin stain; ×300)

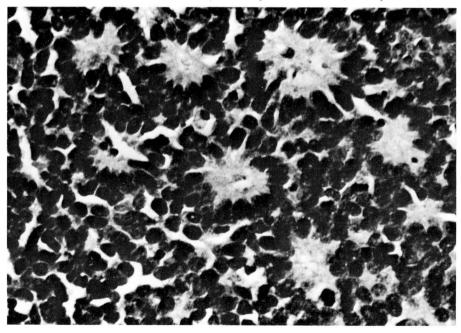

inoblastoma, it may appear as a superficial white retinal mass arising from the nerve fiber layer, and may contain dense calcification. In contrast to retinoblastoma, it is often associated with adenoma sebaceum, seizures, and a family history of tuberous sclerosis. In cases where these findings are absent, however, it may be impossible to differentiate an astrocytoma from a small retinoblastoma by clinical means.

Capillary Hemangioma of the Retina. This tumor is also discussed later in this chapter. Like retinoblastoma, the capillary hemangioma is an autosomal dominant retinal tumor which may be solitary or multiple. The tumor is slightly red or pink, rather than white, does not have calcifications, and is usually associated with deep yellow exudates which may involve the fovea, findings which are also not present with retinoblastoma. The capillary hemangioma is usually diagnosed in older children or young adults, while retinoblastoma usually appears in infancy.

Early Coats' Disease. Retinal telangiectasia with exudation (Coats' disease; see in Chap. 6) may also resemble retinoblastoma. In contrast to retinoblastoma, however, it shows typical aneurysmal dilatation of the vessels, associated with extensive yellow exudation in the periphery and posterior pole. Although Coats' disease does not usually produce a distinct mass, it may be associated with a yellowish white pseudotumor due to organized hemorrhage, fibrosis, and gliosis.[17] It usually occurs unilaterally, it is more common in males, and there is no familial tendency.

Nematode Granuloma. Peripheral granulomas secondary to nematode infestation (see Nematode Endophthalmitis, in Chap. 5) produce a white peripheral mass which can simulate retinoblastoma. Unlike retinoblastoma, however, it is always solitary and unilateral, and often produces a rather severe vitreous reaction with membranes extending from the posterior pole to the periphery. Shrinkage of the lesion may drag the retina and its vessels and produce a retinal fold, a finding which does not occur with retinoblastoma. In difficult cases, aqueous cytology and enzymes, as discussed in Chapter 5, have been used to make the differentiation.[30]

Peripheral Uveoretinitis. Idiopathic peripheral uveoretinitis (see Chap. 5) may also simulate a retinoblastoma by producing a white exudative lesion at the ora serrata and pars plana. In contrast to a small peripheral retinoblastoma, it produces a more severe vitreous reaction with distinct exudation on the pars plana inferiorly. A retinoblastoma may occasionally assume a diffuse growth pattern and more closely resemble peripheral uveoretinitis, but the latter condition is frequently associated with cystoid maculopathy, a finding not present with retinoblastoma.

Retrolental Fibroplasia (Retinopathy of Prematurity). (See Chap. 6.) In advanced stages this condition may produce a total retinal detachment and leukocoria, while in milder cases there may be an organized mass in the temporal periphery that superficially simulates retinoblastoma. In contrast to retinoblastoma, however, retrolental fibroplasia is more likely to be bilateral and symmetrical, and to show tractional phenomena, with dragging of the retina. In addition, most patients have a history of prematurity.

Medulloepithelioma. This tumor is discussed below, under Tumors of the Nonpigmented Ciliary Epithelium.

Organized Hemorrhage. Organized hemorrhage in the peripheral fundus due to trauma or other insults may result in a white fibrous tissue mass with focal nodularity resembling the "cottage cheese" appearance of regressed retinoblastoma. In some cases a history of trauma cannot be elicited and the diagnosis is presumptive.

Diagnostic Techniques

The diagnosis of retinoblastoma can usually be made by means of a good history and an ocular examination using indirect ophthalmoscopy. Unfortunately, most cases are not recognized until the lesion is quite advanced and producing leukocoria. The recognition of small peripheral lesions is best made by examination under anesthesia with careful indirect ophthalmoscopy and gentle scleral depression.

Fluorescein angiography is difficult to perform and not particularly helpful in the diagnosis. Orbital x-rays or ultrasonography may demonstrate calcium in the mass, which is helpful but not pathognomonic.[32] Ultrasonography reveals a normal-sized eye in most cases of retinoblastoma.

Certain laboratory studies aid in diagnosis. The aqueous plasma lactate dehydrogenase (LDH) and phosphoglucose isomerase (PGI) assays have been found helpful by some investigators.[10, 37] Carcinoembryonic antigen (CEA) levels may be elevated in certain patients with retinoblastoma, although the significance of this has not been fully determined.[11, 20]

Treatment

The treatment of retinoblastoma varies with the state of the disease and the philosophy of the physician.[8] Large unilateral lesions which fill most of the globe are usually treated by enucleation. Small lesions are often asymptomatic and located in the only remaining eye. Such lesions are treated with external irradiation, photocoagulation, cobalt plaque application, or cryotherapy, depending upon the extent of involvement.

External irradiation is performed by giving 3500 to 4000 R over a 3-week period, through either an anterior or lateral portal. In a few weeks the lesion usually shows a decrease in size and has a cottage cheese appearance (Fig. 7-6).

Xenon arc photocoagulation is usually performed by placing two rows of treatment in uninvolved retinal tissue around the lesion. In 3 to 4 weeks the same area is treated again. When the retinal blood supply to the tumor is destroyed, the lesion regresses (Fig. 7-7).

Cobalt plaque treatment is done by suturing a Cobalt-60 plaque on the sclera over the base of the tumor. The plaque is left in place for a designated period of time in order to deliver 3500 to 4000 R to the tumor apex. The plaque is then removed surgically. The desired result is a regression pattern similar to

(Text continues on page 146.)

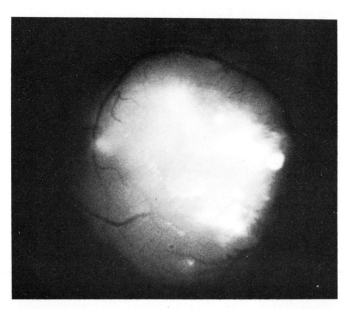

FIG. 7-6. Fundus photogr
of a regressed retinoblast
following external beam
irradiation.

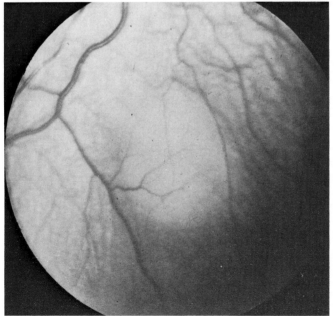

FIG. 7-7. A. Fundus
photograph of a small
retinoblastoma below the
optic disc.
Continued opposite page.

A

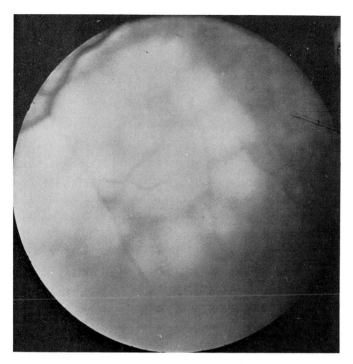

FIG. 7-7. *Continued.* **B.** Same lesion immediately after surrounding xenon photo-coagulation. **C.** Same lesion 3 weeks later, showing disappearance of the tumor, leaving a depressed chorioretinal scar.

B

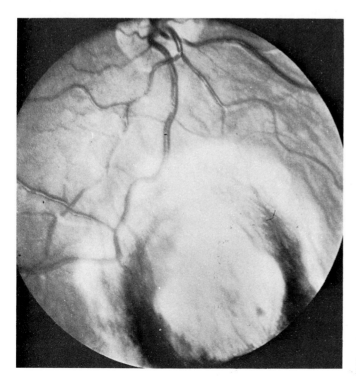

C

that seen with external irradiation (Fig. 7-8). Cobalt plaque therapy may be used as a primary procedure or in cases where other treatment modalities have failed.

Cryotherapy is done by freezing around and over the base of the lesion with a transscleral approach. Once the blood supply to the tumor is destroyed, a regression pattern occurs that is similar to that seen with photocoagulation.

ASTROCYTOMA

The astrocytoma (astrocytic hamartoma) of the retina appears clinically as one or more white masses located anywhere in the fundus. It occurs in two forms. One is a smooth, slightly elevated superficial white mass located in the nerve fiber layer of the retina. The other is a more densely compact mass with calcified nodules resembling fish eggs. (Plate 2, C). The tumor is nonprogressive or very slowly progressive and in most cases does not cause marked ocular symptoms. It is associated with tuberous sclerosis or (Bourneville's disease), characterized by mental retardation, seizures, and similar hamartomas in the brain, kidney, heart, or other organs.[13] Identical retinal tumors are seen in patients with neurofibromatosis and sometimes in patients who are otherwise normal. The differentiation of astrocytoma from retinoblastoma is discussed above, under Retinoblastoma.

Histologically, the retinal astrocytic hamartoma is usually confined to the nerve fiber layer, although large tumors may replace the inner half of the sensory retina (Fig. 7-9). The tumor is composed of well-differentiated fibrillar astrocytes with round nuclei. Foci of calcification are often present within the tumor.

Treatment of an astrocytic hamartoma of the retina is not usually necessary. Most cases remain stationary for years and show no sifnificant progression.

CAPILLARY HEMANGIOMA

The capillary hemangioma, (Plate 2, D), occurs as one or more red or pink masses which may be located anywhere in the fundus. It is first seen most often in older children or young adults. The classic features include a dilated tortuous afferent retinal artery and an efferent retinal vein. Yellow exudation in the outer retinal layers may progressively accumulate, leading to an exudative retinal detachment. This exudate may preferentially accumulate in the posterior pole remote from the tumor itself, producing a stellate macular exudate.

The capillary hemangioma of the retina is classically recognized as a part of von Hippel-Lindau disease, an autosomal dominant condition with incomplete penetrance. Patients with this condition classically have retinal and cerebellar hemangiomas, often associated with hamartomas of multiple organs, including pheochromocytomas, hypernephromas, pancreatic cysts, and epididymal or ovarian cysts.

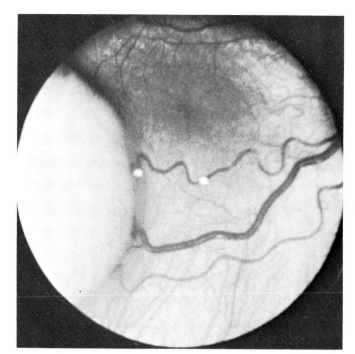

FIG. 7-8. A. Fundus photograph of a small retinoblastoma temporal to the macula. **B.** Same lesion 3 weeks after Cobalt-60 plaque therapy, showing marked regression of the tumor.

A

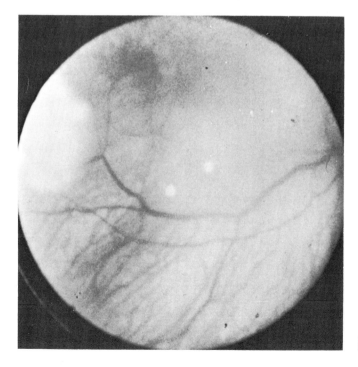

B

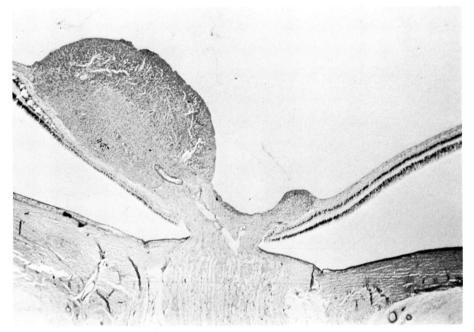

FIG. 7-9. Low-power photomicrograph of an astrocytic hamartoma near the optic disc. (AFIP accession no. 219942) (Hematoxylin-eosin stain; ×10)

Histologically, the capillary hemangioma of the retina consists of a benign proliferation of endothelial cells of the retinal capillaries (Fig. 7-10). Variable numbers of clear astrocytes may also be present. The tumor arises from the nerve fiber layer of the retina.

The treatment of the retinal capillary hemangioma includes photocoagulation, cryotherapy, or diathermy with a scleral buckling procedure, depending on the size and extent of the tumor.[1]

CAVERNOUS HEMANGIOMA

Cavernous hemangioma of the retina (Fig. 7-11) may vary from a few small venous aneurysms to a large group of aneurysms which resemble a cluster of grapes. This tumor is often associated with similar vascular hamartomas of the skin and central nervous system.[15] Fluorescein angiography shows very characteristic features in retinal cavernous hemangioma. The vascular spaces are hypofluorescent in the early angiograms and exhibit slowly progressive accumulation of dye. In the late angiograms there is a typical fluorescein–blood interface, with hyperfluorescence of the superior portion and hypofluorescence of the inferior portion of the vascular spaces.[15]

Treatment is not usually necessary for cavernous hemangioma of the retina. Most lesions are asymptomatic and the only complication is an infrequently occurring vitreous hemorrhage.

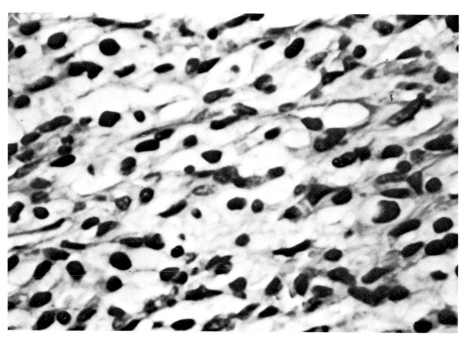

FIG. 7-10. Photomicrograph of a capillary hemangioma of the retina. (AFIP accession no. 301671) (Hematoxylin-eosin stain; ×300)

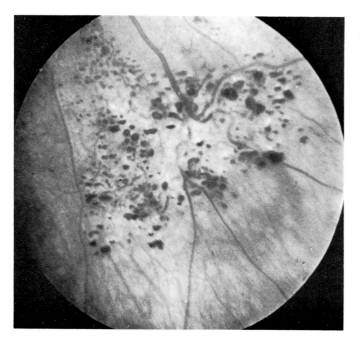

FIG. 7-11. Fundus photograph of a cavernous hemangioma of the retina.

TUMORS OF THE NONPIGMENTED CILIARY EPITHELIUM

Tumors of the nonpigmented ciliary epithelium (pars ciliaris retinae) are rare. They are usually benign, although malignant lesions have been observed. Certain benign tumors may be locally invasive, causing extensive destruction to the globe.

Zimmerman has classified tumors of the ciliary epithelium into two groups.[40] The congenital group consists of glioneuroma, medulloepithelioma and teratoid medulloepithelioma. The acquired group consists of pseudo-epitheliomatous hyperplasia (Fuchs' "adenoma"), adenoma, and adenocarcinoma.

GLIONEUROMA

Glioneuroma, an extremely rare congenital tumor, is characterized by replacement of a large part of the anterior segment by well-differentiated brain tissue containing both neurons and glial cells.

MEDULLOEPITHELIOMA

This tumor, previously called a diktyoma, may occur in either a benign or a malignant form. The tumor usually occurs in young children, but occasionally is first recognized at a later age. The family history is negative. Although it is usually a localized fleshy mass, the tumor may become cystic, and large cysts may float freely in the anterior chamber. The lesion usually grows very slowly and may produce a subluxated lens, glaucoma, retinal detachment, and other complications. In some cases the tumor fills the entire globe, but systemic metastasis, even from those which are cytologically malignant, is extremely rare.

The differential diagnosis of medulloepithelioma includes retinoblastoma, malignant melanoma, and other ciliary body tumors. If the lesion has the typical characteristics just described, the diagnosis is not particularly difficult. In other cases, however, the differentiation may be virtually impossible. The fact that it rarely involves the posterior segment, often has large cysts, and is unilateral helps to distinguish it from retinoblastoma.

Histologically, the medulloepithelioma arises from the nonpigmented ciliary epithelium. It is characterized by convoluted cords of cells which resemble primitive medulloepithelium. The cellular bands appear polarized, and show a fenestrated membrane corresponding to the external limiting membrane.

TERATOID MEDULLOEPITHELIOMA

This extremely rare tumor is clinically similar to other medulloepitheliomas, but histologically it contains heteroplastic elements such as hyaline cartilage, brain tissue, and skeletal muscle.[40]

PSEUDOEPITHELIOMATOUS HYPERPLASIA (FUCHS' "ADENOMA")

Pseudoepitheliomatous hyperplasia is rarely seen clinically but it is commonly observed post mortem or in enucleated eyes. It appears as a white focal mass which is usually located in the pars plicata. Its incidence progressively increases with age.[18] Histologically, it consists of a mass of homogeneous eosinophilic basement membrane material, presumably elaborated by the ciliary epithelium.

ADENOMA AND ADENOCARCINOMA

These tumors of the nonpigmented ciliary epithelium are extremely rare and are often impossible to differentiate clinically from an amelanotic melanoma of the ciliary body. Like melanomas, these tumors have been known to show progressive enlargement, to produce a subluxated lens, and to demonstrate extrascleral extension.

TUMORS OF THE PIGMENT EPITHELIUM

True neoplasms of the pigment epithelium are extremely rare. The pigment epithelium has a peculiar tendency, however, to undergo hyperplasia, or proliferation, which commonly results in a lesion that may resemble a melanoma or other pigmented tumor. In addition, certain congenital abnormalities are known to involve the pigment epithelium in the peripheral fundus.

CONGENITAL HYPERTROPHY

This condition is discussed in Chapter 4. It is mentioned here because it frequently closely resembles a pigmented tumor of the periphery. In contrast to true tumors, it is not elevated and is nonprogressive.

REACTIVE HYPERPLASIA

As previously mentioned, the pigmented epithelium has a tendency to undergo nonneoplastic proliferation, or hyperplasia. This is likely to occur following ocular trauma or inflammation.[28] The resultant mass (Fig. 7-12) may closely resemble a malignant melanoma. In contrast to melanoma, however, it is usually jet black, has an irregular margin, and is rapidly progressive. The involved eye may show other evidence of previous trauma or inflammation, and the patient will usually confirm this history.

Histologically, the hyperplasia consists of cords of pigment epithelium, often with large amounts of eosinophilic basement membrane material.

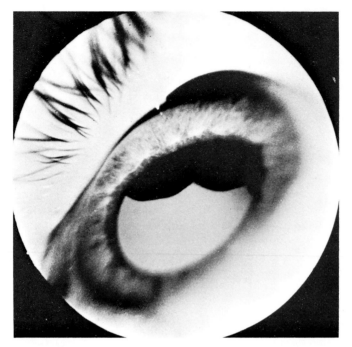

A

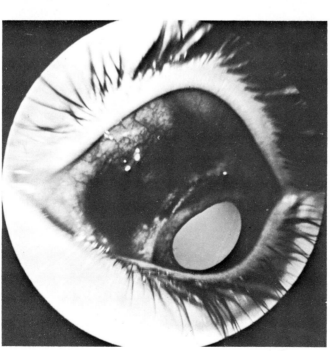

B

FIG. 7-12. A. Pigmented intraocular mass seconda to a presumed reactive proliferation of the retina pigment epithelium. **B.** Episcleral pigmentation i the same eye. (Shields JA et al.: Arch Ophthalmol 89:519–522, 1973)

COMBINED HAMARTOMA

This rather unusual tumor is believed to be a congenital condition which, though present at birth, may not be clinically diagnosed until late childhood or adult life. It classically occurs near the optic disc but may also occur in the fundus periphery.[16]

The peripheral tumor is characterized by a slate gray mass near the equator. It may superficially resemble a large choroidal nevus or a small melanoma but, in contrast to these, it is associated with vitreoretinal traction that often drags the sensory retina in the direction of the mass.

Although the histology of the peripheral lesion has not been studied, it is probably identical to the histology of the same lesion in the posterior pole. This consists of a proliferation of retinal pigment epithelium, small blood vessels, and glial cells. It is probably the contraction of the glial cells that accounts for the retinal traction observed clinically.

ADENOMA

Adenomas or epitheliomas of the peripheral pigment epithelium are rather rare. Although they are benign, they may be impossible to differentiate from malignant melanoma of the uveal tract. Most cases on record have been enucleated as suspected melanomas.[9] Ancillary studies such as fluorescein angiography, ultrasonography, and the ^{32}P test (see Chap. 2) are not helpful in differentiating this lesion from melanoma. The tumor may progressively enlarge and produce a subluxated lens, invasion of the anterior chamber angle, and secondary glaucoma.

Histologically, this tumor consists of a benign proliferation of well-differentiated pigment epithelial cells which form cords. Clear vacuoles are frequently present in the mass.

ADENOCARCINOMA

Malignant tumors arising from the peripheral pigment epithelium are extremely rare and only a few cases have been recorded. Although the tumor may be locally invasive, distant metastasis is unlikely. Clinically the tumor is probably impossible to differentiate from malignant melanoma.

TUMORS OF THE UVEAL TRACT

CHOROIDAL NEVUS

The choroidal nevus is usually asymptomatic and when located in the peripheral fundus it is discovered on routine ophthalmoscopy. Although the vast majority of choroidal nevi are nonprogressive, some occasionally undergo neoplastic change, proliferating into malignant melanoma.

Clinical Features

The choroidal nevus is usually a relatively flat, slate gray lesion with a distinct but feathery margin (Fig. 7-13). It may be as small as ½ disc diameter or as large as 7 or 8 disc diameters. Although it is usually flat, it may attain a thickness of 2 mm. Overlying alterations in the retinal pigment epithelium—drusen, orange pigment, and occasionally a small serous detachment of the sensory retina—may occur.[21]

Nevi may produce other effects on the adjacent structures, particularly degeneration of the overlying retinal pigment epithelium, drusen, loss of photoreceptors, and cystic retinal changes. This explains the visual field defect which can often be demonstrated in these cases.

The differential diagnosis of choroidal nevus includes small choroidal melanomas, hypertrophy of the retinal pigment epithelium, and other pigmented lesions. In most cases the lesion is rather typical and differentiation causes little or no problem. Distinguishing a nevus from a melanoma is discussed under differential diagnosis of malignant melanoma.

Pathology

The histopathology of the choroidal nevus varies. The cells are predominantly densely packed spindle cells, but deeply pigmented plump to polyhedral cells may occasionally be present. If the tumor is composed exclusively

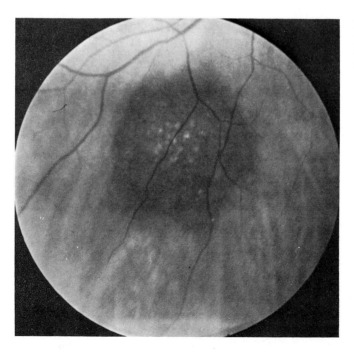

FIG. 7-13. Fundus photograph of a choroidal nevus with overlying drusen.

of these latter cells, it is called a melanocytoma and is identical to the melanocytoma which occurs over the optic disc.

MALIGNANT MELANOMA

Malignant melanoma of the uveal tract is the most common primary intraocular malignancy. It is typically a disease of older adults and is most commonly diagnosed between ages 40 and 70. It shows no predisposition for either sex and it occurs with equal frequency in the right and left eye. Bilateral cases are extremely rare.

In recent years there has been increasing controversy regarding the diagnosis, treatment, and histologic classification of choroidal melanomas.[26] The controversy regarding management is particularly applicable to peripheral melanomas because patients often have reasonably good visual acuity and are reluctant to have enucleation. There are currently several other methods of treatment which are being used for such patients.

Clinical Features

The clinical features of posterior uveal melanomas may vary with their location, depending upon whether they originate in the ciliary body or in the choroid.

Ciliary Body Melanoma. Melanomas arising from the ciliary body often reach a fairly large size before they are recognized clinically. Such tumors may be found on routine examination in an asymptomatic patient when the pupil is widely dilated, allowing visualization of a variably pigmented mass behind the iris (Fig. 7-14). In other cases the patient may become symptomatic, developing lenticular astigmatism owing to compression of the lens equator by the mass. The patient may later develop further visual loss from a sector cataract which is most dense in the quadrant of the tumor.

Certain other clinical signs are also suggestive of ciliary body melanoma. One of the hallmarks is a dilated, often tortuous, episcleral blood vessel in the quadrant of the tumor. Such vessels remain in the same position when the overlying conjunctiva is moved, indicating that they are deep to the conjunctiva. Sometimes a ciliary body melanoma may invade the anterior chamber angle and appear as a dark mass behind the peripheral cornea. The intraocular pressure is usually lower than in the fellow eye. As further infiltration of the angle occurs, acute secondary glaucoma may develop.

A rather ominous sign associated with a ciliary body melanoma is the presence of extraocular extension (Fig. 7-15). This usually appears as one or more pigmented nodules located 3 to 4 mm. posterior to the limbus. Although the extension may resemble an intercalary staphyloma, transillumination will reveal a dark shadow, while a staphyloma will readily transmit light.

Choroidal Melanoma. A peripheral choroidal melanoma is often asymptomatic until it attains a large size. Ophthalmoscopically, there is no

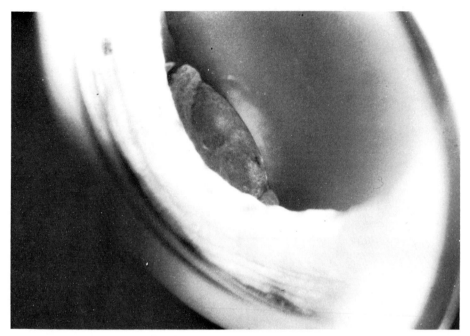

FIG. 7-14. Pigmented malignant melanoma of the ciliary body as seen through the dilated pupil.

FIG. 7-15. Extraocular extension of a malignant melanoma of the peripheral choroid and ciliary body.

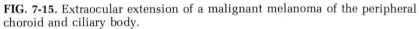

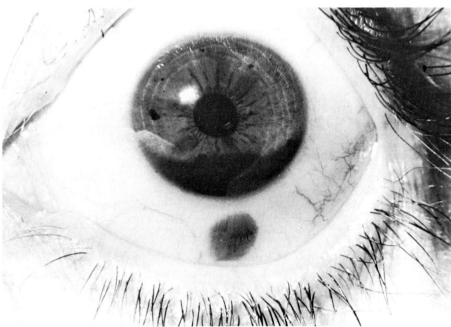

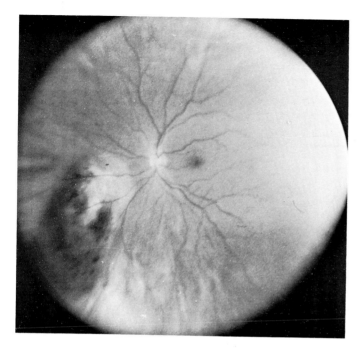

FIG. 7-16. Wide-angle fundus photograph of a malignant melanoma of the choroid in the inferonasal portion of the fundus.

difference between tumors arising in the posterior pole and those in the peripheral choroid.

A small- to medium-sized choroidal melanoma appears as an elevated fundus mass ranging in color from a creamy yellow to dark gray (Fig. 7-16). In contrast to benign nevi, the tumor is usually greater than 5 mm. in diameter and 2 mm. in thickness. It may range from deeply pigmented to amelanotic. Surface changes such as drusen and orange pigment are often pronounced. A serous retinal detachment of variable extent may also be present.

A larger melanoma in the peripheral choroid may extend into the visual axis, causing visual loss (Fig. 7-17). Such tumors may break through Bruch's membrane, producing a mushroom configuration (Fig. 7-18). When this occurs the tumor may show dilated choroidal vessels within the dome of the mass. A large serous retinal detachment may extend to the posterior pole and eventually involve the entire fundus. The subretinal fluid in such cases shows dramatic shifting with movement of the head and may cause secondary glaucoma by producing either rubeosis iridis or anterior displacement of the lens–iris diaphragm.

Pathology

The pathologic features of melanomas of the ciliary body and peripheral choroid are well known. They may be divided into those features observed in the freshly sectioned eye or with low-power microscopy, and the cytologic features observed on high-power microscopy.

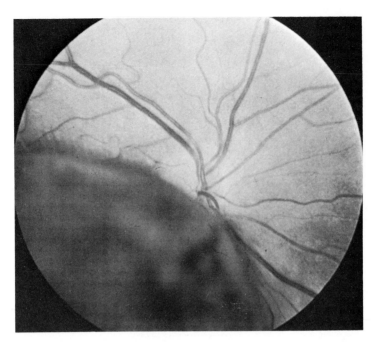

FIG. 7-17. Fundus photograph of a peripheral choroidal melanoma which has extended into the visual axis.

Grossly, melanomas of the peripheral uvea may assume several growth patterns. The smaller tumors may be oval-shaped, but, as mentioned, the larger ones may break through Bruch's membrane and produce the mushroom configuration observed clinically (Figs. 7-18 and 7-19). Such tumors are usually associated with a rather extensive retinal detachment. Peripheral uveal melanomas may show profound microscopic effects upon adjacent ocular structures. Compression upon the lens can produce a focal or complete cataract. The overlying retinal pigment epithelium may show degenerative changes, with drusen and with macrophages containing liberated lipofuscin pigment. The retina may show microcystoid changes which may lead to secondary degenerative retinoschisis (see in Chap. 8).

Classification

Cytologically, uveal melanomas have conventionally been divided into six categories known as the Callender classification.[6] They are (1) spindle A, (2) spindle B, (3) fascicular, (4) mixed, (5) necrotic, and (6) epithelioid. The prognosis following enucleation is better for pure spindle A and spindle B tumors and worse for mixed or pure epithelioid cell tumors.

McLean and co-workers[19] have proposed a new classification which places many of the more benign-appearing spindle A tumors into a category of benign lesions known as spindle cell nevi. They place the more suspicious spindle A tumors with the spindle B type in a separate category known as spindle cell melanomas. This classification will probably become more widely accepted in the future.

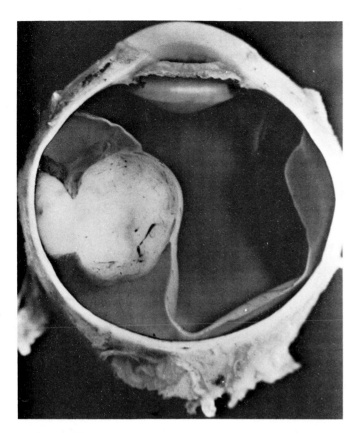

FIG. 7-18. Amelanotic melanoma of the peripheral choroid showing a mushroom-shaped configuration and an overlying serous detachment of the retina.

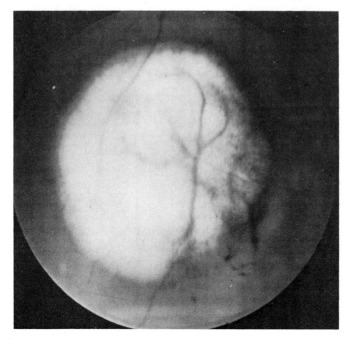

FIG. 7-19. Fundus photograph of the dome of a choroidal melanoma which has broken through Bruch's membrane. Note the large dilated vessels on the surface.

Differential Diagnosis

The differential diagnosis of peripheral uveal melanomas includes many of the same lesions which may resemble melanomas of the posterior pole, as well as some lesions which are unique to the peripheral fundus. For example, lesions often confused with posterior segment melanomas, such as disciform macular degeneration and melanocytoma of the optic disc, are not usually included in the differential diagnosis of peripheral lesions. Some of the more important peripheral fundus lesions which may simulate melanoma will be considered here. Differentiation of degenerative retinoschisis from melanoma is discussed in Chapter 8.

Choroidal Nevus. In many cases it may be clinically impossible to differentiate a large suspicious nevus from a small melanoma. In such cases it is usually safe to monitor the lesion closely for evidence of growth before initiating treatment.

Rhegmatogenous Retinal Detachment. This lesion was the one most often erroneously enucleated as suspected melanoma in two large series of pseudomelanomas reported from the Armed Forces Institute of Pathology.[12, 35] With the widespread use of indirect ophthalmoscopy, the differentiation is easier. The typical rippled appearance of the detachment, with a retinal hole and lack of shifting subretinal fluid, should help in differentiating this lesion from a melanoma.

Choroidal Detachment. Although a peripheral choroidal detachment may resemble a melanoma ophthalmoscopically, the former is usually multilobed and annular, and usually occurs in a hypotonous eye following intraocular surgery. When there is any doubt as to diagnosis, transillumination will demonstrate transmission of light with a choroidal detachment and a shadow with a melanoma. It is important to remember that in some instances a fundus mass which is detected following cataract extraction may be a choroidal melanoma that clinically resembles a choroidal detachment.[29]

Choroidal Effusion Syndrome. A variant of choroidal detachment which may also resemble a peripheral melanoma is the choroidal effusion syndrome. There is usually no history of ocular surgery and the patient presents with a peripheral brown mass associated with a serous retinal detachment and shifting subretinal fluid. The peripheral mass, however, readily transmits light and is more likely to be multilobed and annular.

Peripheral Exudative Hemorrhagic Chorioretinopathy. This condition may closely resemble a peripheral choroidal melanoma. Differentiation between the two is discussed in Chapter 8.

Metastatic Tumor. Tumors metastatic to the choroid may occasionally be confused with a primary choroidal melanoma. The metastatic lesion usually occurs in the posterior pole but may occasionally involve the peripheral choroid and ciliary body. In contrast to melanoma, it is almost always a creamy yellow color with brown pigment clumps on the surface. Pigmentation within the tumor itself is unusual. A history of mastectomy or the discovery of a primary tumor may help in the differentiation. Ultrasonography may also be diagnostically useful in such cases.[36]

Congenital Hypertrophy of the Retinal Pigment Epithelium. When it occurs in the periphery, congenital hypertrophy of the retinal pigment epithelium (see in Chap. 4) tends to be larger and often gives the false impression of elevation. In contrast to melanoma, this lesion is flat, has a well-delineated margin, and is nonprogressive.[22]

Hyperplasia of the Retinal Pigment Epithelium. This condition may closely resemble a malignant melanoma. Differentiating features are discussed under Reactive Hyperplasia, above.

Posterior Scleritis. Posterior scleritis may also resemble a choroidal melanoma.[3] The patient usually has a history of recurrent diffuse anterior scleritis and, sometimes, rheumatoid arthritis. The lesion is more likely to be posterior in the macular area. It is amelanotic and often associated with choroidal folds. There is usually a dramatic response to systemic or retrobulbar corticosteroids.

Choroidal Hemangioma. The choroidal hemangioma is mentioned here for completeness because it may also resemble a choroidal melanoma. Choroidal hemangiomas, however, are usually located in the posterior pole and are rarely a consideration in the differential diagnosis of a peripheral fundus lesion. In contrast to melanoma, the hemangioma has a red-orange color, sometimes hardly distinguishable from the background fundus.

Diagnostic Techniques

A number of procedures are available to aid in the diagnosis of malignant melanoma of the choroid.[26, 31] In eyes with clear media, the indirect ophthalmoscope is the most useful tool. In eyes with opaque media, the indirect ophthalmoscope is not helpful and other techniques are utilized. The ancillary techniques which are most helpful in the diagnosis of choroidal melanoma include transillumination, fluorescein angiography, ultrasonography, and the radioactive phosphorus uptake (^{32}P) test. The basic principles of these techniques are discussed in Chapter 2.

Transillumination. Pigmented choroidal melanomas will completely block the transmission of light, minimally pigmented melanomas will partially block transmission, and amelanotic melanomas will allow transmission of light. The technique is most useful in differentiating a choroidal detachment from a peripheral uveal melanoma.

Fluorescein Angiography. With this technique, melanomas often show a typical, although not diagnostic pattern. Most melanomas show mottled fluorescence during the arterial or venous phases, with progressive staining throughout the angiogram. The pattern will vary greatly with the status of the overlying retinal pigment epithelium. Orange pigment on the tumor surface will block transmission, producing areas of hypofluorescence. Drusen on the surface will permit more transmission of background fluorescence, leading to hyperfluorescence. Pinpoint areas of hyperfluorescence along the tumor margins are often seen in the recirculation phase. They probably represent areas of defective pigment epithelium or cystic spaces which retain the fluorescein.

Ultrasonography. Both A-scan and B-scan ultrasonograms show rather typical patterns with choroidal melanomas. With the B-scan procedure, small to medium-sized melanomas show an oval shape with smooth anterior borders, acoustic hollowness, choroidal excavation, and orbital shadowing. When the tumor breaks through Bruch's membrane, the typical mushroom shape can be detected with the B scan. An A scan shows a high initial spike and low to medium internal reflectivity.

Radioactive Phosphorus Uptake (^{32}P) Test. Although this procedure has been somewhat controversial, we have found it to be highly accurate for differentiating choroidal melanoma from benign lesions which simulate melanoma.[27] If the suspected lesion is in the ciliary body, the test can be performed without surgery. If the lesion is centered at or posterior to the equator, it is usually necessary to do a peritomy to gain access to it.[34]

There are certain situations in which the diagnostic value of the ^{32}P test is limited. The test will not always differentiate a large choroidal nevus from a small chroidal melanoma. The results in such cases may be borderline, leading to difficulty in making a therapeutic decision. The test will also not differentiate an amelanotic melanoma from a metastatic tumor to the choroid, both of which produce positive results.[27]

The ^{32}P test is highly accurate, however, for differentiating melanoma from certain benign fundus lesions. Thus, the result is usually negative for choroidal hemangiomas and disciform macular degeneration, both of which may simulate melanoma.

Treatment

The treatment of choroidal melanomas is controversial. Traditionally, most eyes with such tumors were enucleated soon after the diagnosis was suspected. Recently, the concept of enucleation for choroidal melanomas has been challenged.[41] Patients with peripheral uveal melanomas often have good visual acuity in the involved eye. Consequently, methods of management designed to preserve vision have been utilized.

Observation. There has been an increasing tendency among some authorities to manage some small to medium-sized choroidal melanomas by observation and to reserve treatment for those lesions which show definite evidence of growth. This is particularly true for small tumors which appear dormant or quiescent.

Photocoagulation. This method has been utilized for selected small melanomas, and the indications and technique are described in the literature.[26] The tumor is first surrounded by photocoagulation, and subsequent treatments are directed to the surface of the lesion. The desired result is a flat area of scar tissue overlying the bare sclera.

Radiotherapy. Most choroidal melanomas are not particularly radiosensitive and external beam irradiation is usually ineffective. The method of treatment has therefore been to suture a radiation plaque to the sclera at the base of the tumor. Cobalt-60 has been most widely used. It appears to be most effective for tumors which are actively proliferating, and less effective for melanomas which are stationary or slowly progressive.

Iridocyclectomy. This involves surgical removal of melanomas of the iris root and ciliary body. Several techniques have been developed. Complications such as subluxation of the lens, cataract, and vitreous hemorrhage are rather common, particularly if more than one-fourth of the pars plicata must be resected.

Eye Wall Resection. This technique has been developed for the surgical removal of small to medium-sized choroidal melanomas which are centered in the region of the equator. The preliminary preparation involves the application of photocoagulation or cryotherapy around the tumor; this is followed by a full-thickness resection of all ocular coats in the area of the tumor. The defect is replaced by a scleral graft. Although this technique is often successful, there is usually some degree of visual loss following surgery.

Enucleation. Most large choroidal melanomas are still managed by enucleation, although some authorities have suggested that the trauma or other effects of enucleation may promote the spread of tumor cells.[41] A so-called "no-touch" technique has recently been utilized in order to minimize the possible complications, but its effectiveness is still undetermined.[14]

Exenteration. Exenteration of the orbital contents is recommended by some authorities as the treatment of choice for choroidal or ciliary body melanomas which show significant extrascleral extension. The effectiveness of this technique for preventing metastasis is still uncertain, although one small series indicates that the mortality rate is lower if exenteration is performed in such cases.[25]

TUMOR METASTATIC TO THE UVEA

Tumors metastasizing to the intraocular structures usually involve the uveal tract; metastasis to the retina and the other intraocular structures is rare. Most tumors which are metastatic to the uvea affect the posterior pole, and involvement of the peripheral choroid and ciliary body (see Differential Diagnosis, under Malignant Melanoma) are less common. There appears to be no predilection for either eye, although most studies indicate that the left eye is slightly more commonly involved.

Tumor metastatic to the uvea is a disease of adulthood, being extremely rare in children. It is more common in women than in men because breast carcinoma is the tumor which most commonly metastasizes to the eye. The second most common primary site is the lung, followed by the gastrointestinal tract, kidney, and other organs. Most tumors which are metastatic to the uvea are carcinomas; sarcomas rarely metastasize to the eye. Malignant melanoma of the skin may occasionally spread to the uvea.

Clinical Features

Tumor metastatic to the uvea is an amelanotic irregular lesion which may be flat, placoid, or, less commonly, dome-shaped. In contrast to choroidal melanoma, it is often multifocal or bilateral, particularly when the primary site is the breast. A brown geographic pigmentation on the surface of the tumor (Fig. 7-20) is highly characteristic, but is not always present. An associated retinal detachment is found; its extent is usually greater than one would expect with a choroidal melanoma of comparable size.

Pathologically, the tumor is amelanotic and diffuse or multinodular (Fig. 7-21). The cell type varies with the site of the primary tumor, but in many cases cells are highly undifferentiated.

Ancillary studies such as fluorescein angiography and ultrasonography may be helpful in the diagnosis of metastatic tumors, but they are not always definitive.

Treatment

The treatment of tumors metastatic to the uvea is external beam irradiation, often combined with specific chemotherapy. In advanced cases of breast carcinoma, palliative treatment such as oophorectomy and adrenalectomy may help to control the ocular lesions.

LYMPHOID TUMORS

Although the leukemias may involve the optic nerve, retina, and choroid as part of the widespread disease (see Leukemia, in Chap. 6), it is rather unusual for lymphoid tumors to involve the uveal tract. The two most common lesions are benign reactive lymphoid hyperplasia and certain lymphomas, particularly reticulum cell carcinoma.

BENIGN REACTIVE LYMPHOID HYPERPLASIA

In this condition, the uveal tract, and sometimes the orbit and conjunctiva, are infiltrated by benign lymphocytes and plasma cells.[23] Although the etiology is unknown, there has been some speculation that it may be related to certain dysproteinemias, particularly Waldenström's macroglobulinemia. If the diagnosis can be made clinically, systemic corticosteroids or irradiation is the treatment of choice.

RETICULUM CELL SARCOMA

This condition, a type of lymphoma, may also involve the peripheral choroid and the retina.[2] It often simulates a posterior uveitis with cells in the vitreous. The diagnosis can sometimes be made by cytologic examination of the vitre-

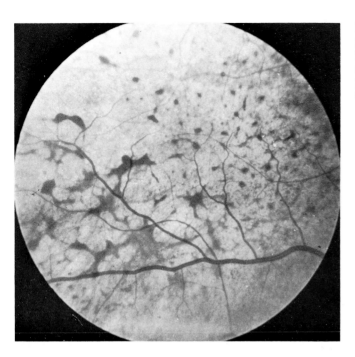

FIG. 7-20. Fundus photograph of the surface of a tumor metastatic to the choroid. Note the typical pigmentation on the surface of the lesion.

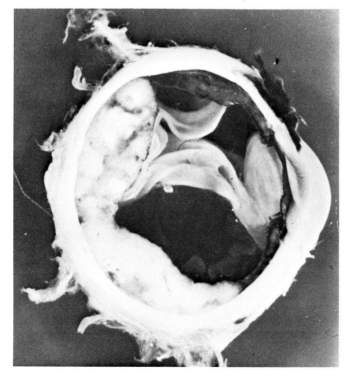

FIG. 7-21. Grossly sectioned globe containing a tumor metastatic to the choroid. Note that the tumor is amelanotic and multinodular, and has produced a large serous detachment of the retina.

ous aspirate, demonstrating the reticulum cells. Once the diagnosis is established, irradiation appears to be the treatment of choice.

REFERENCES

1. **Annesley WH, Leonard BC, Shields JA, Tasman WS:** Fifteen year review of treated cases of retinal angiomatosis. Trans Am Acad Ophthalmol Otolaryngol 83:446–453, 1977
2. **Barr CL, Green WR, Payne JW, Knox DL, Jensen AD, Thompson RL:** Intraocular reticulum cell sarcoma: clinicopathologic study of four cases and review of the literature. Surv Ophthalmol 19:224–239, 1975
3. **Benson WE, Shields JA, Tasman WS, Crandall AE:** Nodular posterior scleritis. Arch Ophthalmol 97:1482–1486, 1979
4. **Bishop JO, Madsen EC:** Retinoblastoma. Review of current status. Surv Ophthalmol 19:342–366, 1975
5. **Boniuk M, Zimmerman LE:** Spontaneous regression of retinoblastoma. Int Ophthalmol Clin 2:525–542, 1962
6. **Callender GR:** Malignant melanotic tumors of the eye: a study of the histologic types in 111 cases. Trans Am Acad Ophthalmol Otolaryngol 36:131–142, 1931
7. **Devesa SS:** The incidence of retinoblastoma. Am J Ophthalmol 80:263–265, 1975
8. **Ellsworth RM:** The practical management of retinoblastoma. Trans Am Ophthalmol Soc 67:462–534, 1969
9. **Fair JR:** Tumors of the retinal pigment epithelium. Am J Ophthalmol 45:495–505, 1958
10. **Felberg NT, McFall R, Shields JA:** Aqueous humor enzyme patterns in retinoblastoma. Invest Ophthalmol 16:1039–1046, 1977
11. **Felberg NT, Michelson JB, Shields JA:** CEA family syndrome: abnormal carcinoembryonic antigen levels in asymptomatic retinoblastoma family members. Cancer 37:1397–1402, 1976
12. **Ferry AP:** Lesion mistaken for malignant melanoma of the posterior uvea. Arch Ophthalmol 72:463–469, 1964
13. **Font RL, Ferry AP:** The phakomatoses. Int Ophthalmol Clin 12:1–50, 1972
14. **Fraunfelder FT, Boozman FW, Wilson RS, Thomas AH:** No-touch technique for intraocular malignant melanoma. Arch Ophthalmol 95:1616–1620, 1977
15. **Gass JDM:** Cavernous hemangioma of the retina. Am J Ophthalmol 71:799–814, 1971
16. **Gass JDM:** An unusual hamartoma of the pigment epithelium and retina simulating choroidal melanoma. Trans Am Ophthalmol Soc 51:171–185, 1973
17. **Green WR:** Bilateral Coats' disease. Arch Ophthalmol 77:378–383, 1967
18. **Iliff WH, Green WR:** Incidence and histology of Fuch's adenoma. Arch Ophthalmol 88:249–254, 1977
19. **McLean IW, Zimmerman LE, Evans RM:** Re-appraisal of Callender's spindle A type of malignant melanoma of the choroid and ciliary body. Am J Ophthalmol 86:557–564, 1978
20. **Michelson JB, Felberg NT, Shields JA:** Carcinoembryonic antigen. Its role in the evaluation of intraocular malignant tumors. Arch Ophthalmol 94:414–416, 1976
21. **Pro M, Shields JA, Tomer TL:** Serous detachment of the fovea associated with presumed choroidal nevi. Arch Ophthalmol 96:1374–1377, 1978
22. **Purcell JJ, Shields JA:** Hypertrophy with hyperpigmentation of the retinal pigment epithelium. Arch Ophthalmol 93:1122–1126, 1975
23. **Ryan SJ, Zimmerman LE, King FM:** Reactive lymphoid hyperplasia. An unusual form of intraocular pseudotumor. Trans Am Acad Ophthalmol Otolaryngol 76:652–671, 1972
24. **Sarin LK, Shields JA:** The differential diagnosis of leukocoria. In Harley RD (ed): Pediatric Ophthalmology. Philadelphia, Saunders, 1975
25. **Shammas HF, Blodi FC:** Orbital extension of choroidal and ciliary body melanomas. Arch Ophthalmol 95:2002–2005, 1977
26. **Shields JA:** Current approaches to the diagnosis and management of choroidal melanomas. Surv Ophthalmol 21:443–463, 1977
27. **Shields JA:** Accuracy and limitation of the ^{32}P test in the diagnosis of ocular tumors. An analysis of 500 cases. Ophthalmology 85:950–966, 1978
28. **Shields JA, Green WR, McDonald PR:** Uveal pseudomelanoma due to post-traumatic pigmentary migration. Arch Ophthalmol 89:519–522, 1973

29. **Shields JA, Leonard BC, Sarin LK:** Multilobed uveal melanoma masquerading as a post-operative choroidal detachment. Br J Ophthalmol 60:386–389, 1976

30. **Shields JA, Lerner HA, Felberg NT:** Aqueous cytology and enzymes in nematode endophthalmitis. Am J Ophthalmol 84:319–322, 1977

31. **Shields JA, McDonald PR:** Improvements in the diagnosis of posterior uveal melanomas. Arch Ophthalmol 91:259–264, 1974

32. **Shields JA, Michelson JB, Leonard BC, Sarin LK:** B-scan ultrasonography in the diagnosis of atypical retinoblastomas. Can J Ophthalmol 11:42–51, 1976

33. **Shields JA, Michelson JB, Leonard BC, Thompson RL:** Retinoblastoma in an 18 year-old male. J Pediatr Ophthalmol 13:274–277, 1976

34. **Shields JA, Sarin LK, Federman JL, Mensheha manhart O, Carmichael PL:** Surgical approach to the ^{32}P test for posterior uveal melanomas. Ophthalmic Surg 5:13–19, 1974

35. **Shields JA, Zimmerman LE:** Lesions simulating malignant melanoma of the posterior uvea. Arch Ophthalmol 89:466–471, 1973

36. **Stephens R, Shields JA:** Diagnosis and management of cancer metastatic to the uvea. A study of 70 cases. Ophthalmology (in press)

37. **Swartz M, Herbst R, Goldberg MF:** Aqueous humor lactic dehydrogenase in retinoblastoma. Am J Ophthalmol 78:612–617, 1974

38. **Ts'o MOM, Fine BS, Zimmerman LE:** The Flexner-Wintersteiner rosettes in retinoblastoma. Arch Pathol Lab Med 88:664–671, 1969

39. **Ts'o MOM, Zimmerman LE, Fine BS:** The nature of retinoblastoma. I. Photoreceptor differentiation. A clinical and histopathological study. Am J Ophthalmol 69:339–349, 1970

40. **Zimmerman LE:** Verhoeff's "terato-neuroma." A critical reappraisal in light of new observations and current concepts of embryonic tumors. Trans Am Ophthalmol Soc 69:210–236, 1971

41. **Zimmerman LE, McLean IW, Foster WD:** Does enucleation of the eye containing a malignant melanoma prevent or accelerate the dissemination of tumor cells? Br J Ophthalmol 62:420–425, 1978

8

Degenerative Conditions

Degenerative conditions of the retina and choroid comprise an important group of fundus diseases. In contrast to dystrophies (see Chap. 3), which are usually bilateral and symmetrical, and have a hereditary pattern, the degenerations are not necessarily bilateral or symmetrical and usually do not have a hereditary tendency.

This chapter will consider degenerative conditions which involve the peripheral retina, uveal tract, and vitreous. These include the cystic degenerations, retinoschisis, paving stone degeneration, lattice degeneration, peripheral exudative hemorrhagic chorioretinopathy, and certain alterations which occur secondary to vitreous or zonular traction.

In addition to the rather specific entities discussed in this chapter, a number of other types of peripheral chorioretinal degenerations are known to occur. Many of these are related to posterior vitreous detachment and conditions discussed in other chapters.

PARS PLANA CYSTS

Cysts of the pars plana region (Fig. 8-1; see also in Chap. 1) are difficult to observe clinically and are only detected by indirect ophthalmoscopy and scleral depression with the pupil widely dilated. They are observed quite commonly in autopsy eyes and have characteristic features when studied with the dissecting microscope.

Clinical Features

Pars plana cysts are typically clear, round to oval structures which are confined to the pars plana and do not extend into the pars plicata or the peripheral retina. They are frequently confined to one ora bay posteriorly, being situated between the dentate processes. These cysts are not usually accompanied by other pathologic changes, although they are commonly observed in association with malignant melanoma of the peripheral choroid and pars plana region. Some authorities believe that pars plana cysts occur more frequently in cases of multiple myeloma and other dysproteinemic states. This matter will be considered in more detail under Clinical Significance.

Pathology

By light microscopy, pars plana cysts appear to be a separation of the nonpigmented from the pigmented ciliary epithelium (Fig. 8-2). The cyst appears clear with hematoxylin-eosin stain, but is positive with alcian blue and other stains for acid mucopolysaccharides. The staining reaction disappears after digestion with hyaluronidase. The presence of this hyaluronidase-sensitive acid mucopolysaccharide suggests that the fluid within the cyst, like vitreous, is elaborated by the nonpigmented ciliary epithelium.

Some pars plana cysts have a tendency to turn milky white after fixation

FIG. 8-1. Ciliary body in a grossly sectioned globe, showing multiple cysts in the pars plana.

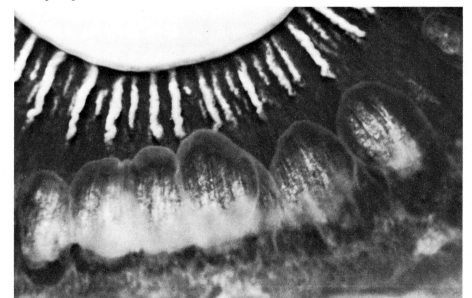

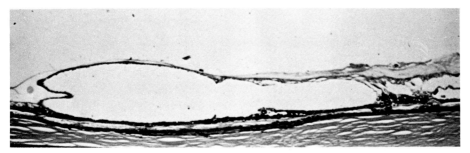

FIG. 8-2. Low-power photomicrograph showing the histology of a pars plana cyst (AFIP accession no. 104874) (Hematoxylin-eosin stain; ×15).

in formalin. Such cysts also stain positively with the periodic acid–Schiff reaction (PAS), and are known to have a high protein content.

Clinical Significance

Most pars plana cysts are found on routine ophthalmologic examination or in postmortem eyes, and apparently have no known clinical significance. At one time there was considerable controversy about the significance of the opaque cysts which are frequently observed in postmortem eyes. Because these are commonly observed in eyes of patients with multiple myeloma, some investigators believed that they were highly suggestive, if not pathognomonic, of that entity. It was later shown, however, that the opacity of the cysts was actually an artifact (albeit a meaningful artifact) of fixation of the eye in formalin, and that the seemingly opaque cysts were actually clear in vivo.[4]

MICROCYSTOID DEGENERATION

Microcystoid degeneration is an extremely common change in the peripheral retina, present to some degree in almost all adult eyes. Like pars plana cysts, this condition is not well appreciated clinically, but is easily observed in enucleated or postmortem eyes.

Clinical Features

Ophthalmoscopically, peripheral microcystoid degeneration appears as a gray band or zone just posterior to the ora serrata. The gray discoloration usually begins in the bases of the dentate processes and gradually coalesces, eventually to involve the entire peripheral retina. The condition is somewhat more pronounced on the temporal side and may be inconspicuous nasally.

The gray appearance often stops at the posterior attachment of the vitreous base, although in some cases it extends behind the equator. The more posterior portions may show white lines, producing a reticulated appearance.

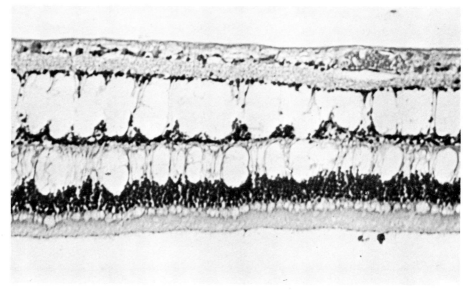

FIG. 8-3. Low-power photomicrograph of peripheral cystoid degeneration of the retina. (AFIP accession no. 1246807) (Hematoxylin-eosin stain; ×40).

Tracing these white lines shows them to be continuous with the retinal vessels. Cystoid degeneration appears to be worse in older patients, in myopes, and in patients with other vitreoretinal disorders.

In the majority of cases peripheral cystoid degeneration is stable, asymptomatic, and nonprogressive. Its only clinical significance is that in rare instances the cysts may continue to coalesce, leading to retinoschisis.

Pathology

In the earliest stages, small clear spaces are present in the outer plexiform layer. These gradually encroach upon the outer layers of the sensory retina (Fig. 8-3). In the most advanced form, the full thickness of the sensory retina is replaced with large cysts which begin to coalesce and form broad areas of splitting in the peripheral retina.

Histologically, peripheral cystoid degeneration is more pronounced on the temporal side than on the nasal side. This factor is used by the ophthalmic pathologist for orientation, because in horizontally sectioned eyes the more advanced cystoid degeneration will invariably be located temporally.

DEGENERATIVE RETINOSCHISIS

Degenerative, or senile, retinoschisis is a sequela of progressive microcystoid degeneration of the peripheral retina. In most cases it is asymptomatic and has little clinical significance, but in rare instances it can progress to retinal detachment.

Clinical Features

Degenerative retinoschisis is a bilateral, often symmetrical condition, which follows coalescence of the intraretinal microcysts seen with peripheral microcystoid degeneration of the retina. It occurs in a relatively flat form or as a bullous elevation.[9] In either case, the lesion usually first appears in the inferotemporal quadrant and may be slowly progressive.

The flat type of retinoschisis looks like an exaggeration of microcystoid degeneration of the peripheral retina. It appears as a broad gray band between the ora serrata and the equator, and rarely progresses posterior to the equator. The cavity itself may be difficult to visualize ophthalmoscopically and is better appreciated by careful examination with the peripheral mirror of the three-mirror contact lens.

The bullous type of retinoschisis has greater clinical significance.[1] It appears clinically as a thin elevated layer of tissue, best observed in the inferotemporal periphery (Plate 3, *A*). The retinal vessels, which often appear white, may be seen passing within this layer, and their shadows may be observed on the background fundus. The thin inner layer of retinoschisis may also show fine white spots on the inner surface (Fig. 8-4 A). With the three-mirror contact lens, multiple small holes may be seen in the inner layer. The fluid within the schisis cavity appears clear.

The outer layer of the schisis cavity, adjacent to the retinal pigment epithelium, also has characteristic features. It has a reddish brown, mottled appearance. Holes in the outer layer are quite different from those in the inner layer. They are large, well delineated, and often have a rolled margin (Fig. 8-4 B). A small rim of fluid, located between the outer layer and the retinal pigment epithelium, may occasionally be present. Pigmented demarcation lines are not a feature of bullous retinoschisis but indicate long-standing retinal detachment.

Significant complications of retinoschisis are rare and only occur with the bullous type.[1] The two major complications are retinal detachment and progression towards the posterior pole, producing an absolute field defect.

Retinal detachment occurs when there are holes in the outer layer of the schisis. In many cases inner layer holes also occur, but they need not be present for retinal detachment to develop. The detachment begins around the outer layer hole and may gradually progress to extend beyond the area of the retinoschisis itself. In an advanced stage it may closely resemble a typical rhegmatogenous detachment secondary to vitreous traction. It has been estimated that about 3 percent of rhegmatogenous retinal detachments occur secondary to holes in the outer layer of a retinoschisis.[3]

When progression towards the posterior pole extends posterior to the equator, perimetry will reveal an absolute field defect. Although clinicians fear that bullous retinoschisis may continue posteriorly to involve the foveal area, this appears to be extremely rare. In some instances, however, there has been foveal involvement, with outer layer holes in the macular region.

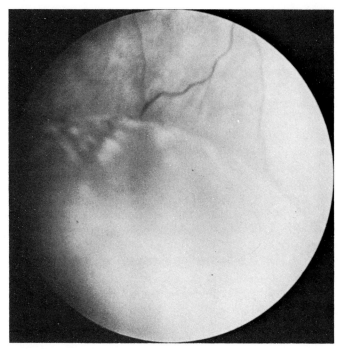

A

FIG. 8-4. A. Frosting in t
inner layer of bullous
retinoschisis. **B.** Outer la
breaks in bullous
retinoschisis. **C.** *Opposite
page.* Low-power
photomicrograph of
degenerative retinoschisi.
(AFIP accession no. 9085
(Hematoxylin-eosin ×40)

B

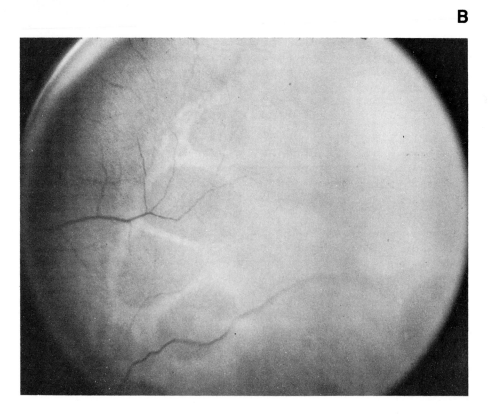

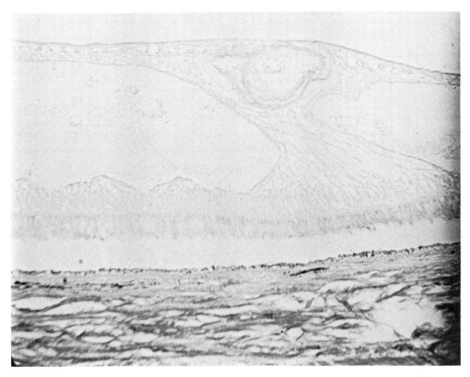

C

Pathology

Since degenerative retinoschisis results from coalescence of the intraretinal microcysts of peripheral cystoid degeneration, the split is usually located in the outer plexiform layers (Fig. 8-4 C). By light microscopy, the retinoschisis cavity appears clear. Remnants of Muller's cells and interrupted axons are often present on both the inner and outer surfaces of the schisis cavity. These correspond to the white dots seen clinically. The walls of the retinal vessels in the inner layer often have a thickening of the fibrous tissue, corresponding to the white lines seen clinically. The vessels are not occluded but are patent, with lumina at least of the caliber of the normal retinal vessels. The outer layer holes have smooth rounded edges which are often rolled over.

Differential Diagnosis

Degenerative retinoschisis may be clinically similar to a number of other fundus conditions. The most important entities in the differential diagnosis are rhegmatogenous retinal detachment, malignant melanoma of the choroid, and juvenile (X-linked) retinoschisis.

Rhegmatogenous retinal detachment (see in Chap. 9) differs from retinoschisis in its rippled rather than smooth appearance. Moreover, it has a horseshoe or round retinal hole and is less likely than retinoschisis to be bilateral and symmetrical. The visual field defect with a retinal detachment is a relative one, whereas the defect with retinoschisis is absolute.

Malignant melanoma of the choroid (see Chap. 7) may also resemble retinoschisis, and eyes with retinoschisis have occasionally been enucleated. In contrast to melanoma, retinoschisis has yellowish white tissue representing remnants of Muller's cells and visual cells on its inner surface. In addition, retinoschisis is bilateral and transmits light with transillumination. Finally, ultrasonography will detect its cystic rather than solid nature.

Juvenile X-linked retinoschisis, a sex-linked recessive disorder, which occurs only in males (see in Chap. 3), should not be confused with degenerative retinoschisis. It is characterized by vitreous veils, stellate macular changes, and frequently by vitreous hemorrhage, findings rarely observed in degenerative retinoschisis.

Treatment

Since most cases of retinoschisis are stationary and asymptomatic, treatment is not usually necessary. If there are outer layer holes with evidence of subretinal fluid, photocoagulation directed to the margins of the holes may be effective in preventing a retinal detachment. If a large retinal detachment has occurred, it should be treated with conventional retinal detachment surgery.

In some cases, photocoagulation or cryotherapy has been used to cause a "collapse" of the schisis cavity. There is no good evidence that such treatment is necessary or helpful. Some authorities have also tried delimiting photocoagulation to prevent the retinoschisis from reaching the macular area. Since progression to the posterior is extremely rare, such treatment is not usually necessary.

PAVING STONE DEGENERATION

Paving stone degeneration, sometimes called cobblestone degeneration, is a chronic, slowly progressive disorder which usually does not produce any symptoms or complications. Its clinical significance lies in the need to differentiate it from other peripheral disorders which have greater clinical importance. Paving stone degeneration is more commonly seen in later years and is bilateral in one-third of the cases.[6]

Clinical Features

Paving stone degeneration is characterized by well-delineated, flat yellow foci ranging from ½ to 2 disc diameters in size. Irregular black pigmentation is frequently present on the margins of the lesions and red lines corresponding to retinal or choroidal blood vessels may traverse them. With time the individual lesions may become confluent and form a continuous band of irregular pigment clumping (Fig. 8-5). Although paving stone degeneration may be located in any quadrant, it is most common and most pronounced inferiorly between the equator and the ora serrata (Fig. 8-6).

Pathology

Light microscopy reveals extensive degeneration of the choroid and the retina (Fig. 8-7). Although the larger choroidal vessels may be present and patent, they are usually sparse. In the area of paving stone degeneration, the choriocapillaris is replaced by loose fibrous connective tissue. Bruch's membrane and the retinal pigment epithelium are attenuated or absent, and there are firm adhesions between the retina and the choroid at that level. The retinal pigment epithelium is often clumped at the margin of the lesion. The retina itself is attenuated and degenerated, with loss of its lamellar architecture. The overlying vitreous is usually normal.

Pathogenesis

Knowledge of the normal choroidal vascular pattern and the histopathology of paving stone degeneration contribute to the understanding of the pathogenesis of this condition. Each lesion of paving stone degeneration is approximately the size of the capillary system supplied by one choroidal artery. Obliteration of the choriocapillaris in the area of the lesion suggests that this condition occurs secondary to progressive occlusion of the precapil-

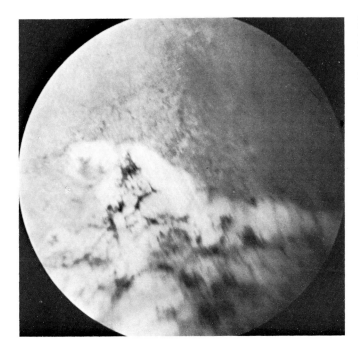

FIG. 8-5. Fundus photograph showing paving stone degeneration near the inferior equator.

lary choroidal arterioles. This results in ischemia in the overlying structures and leads to degeneration of Bruch's membrane, the pigment epithelium, and the sensory retina.

Differential Diagnosis

Several fundus conditions may resemble paving stone degeneration. The most important of these are inactive toxoplasmic retinochoroiditis, lattice degeneration, and retinal holes.

Toxoplasmosis is discussed with the other inflammatory diseases in Chapter 5. Inactive toxoplasmic retinochoroiditis may resemble paving stone degeneration. This condition, however, is more likely to show lesions of more variable size and shape, with posterior pole involvement and overlying vitreous changes.

Lattice degeneration, which will be discussed shortly, also occurs in the peripheral retina. In contrast to paving stone degeneration, it is more common

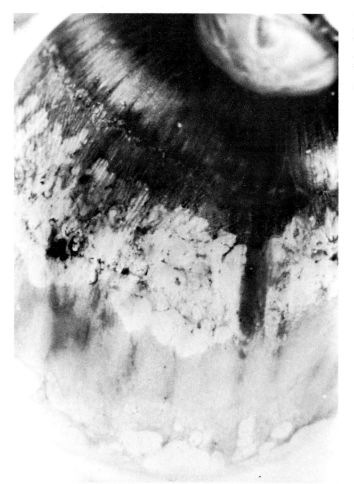

FIG. 8-6. Close-up photograph of a grossly sectioned globe showing paving stone degeneration between the equator and ora serrata.

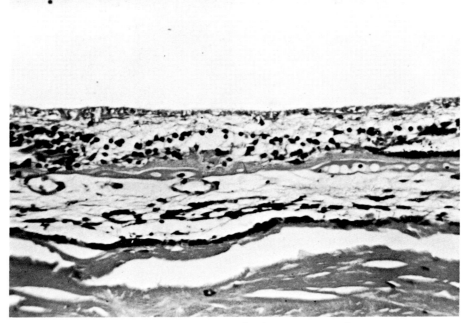

FIG. 8-7. Low-power photomicrograph of paving stone degeneration. (AFIP accession no. 1321857) (Hematoxylin-eosin stain; ×20)

superiorly and is more likely to be equatorial, rather than adjacent to the ora serrata. Its typical appearance should lead to little confusion with paving stone degeneration.

Round retinal holes may resemble focal areas of paving stone degeneration. The yellow appearance of the latter condition, with its traversing blood vessels and absence of subretinal fluid, should differentiate it from a retinal hole. When the focal areas become confluent and lead to the typical paving stone appearance, there should be little diagnostic problem.

LATTICE DEGENERATION

In contrast to the degenerations previously described, lattice degeneration (also known as palisade or equatorial degeneration) has greater clinical significance.[10] It is especially important because of its relationship to rhegmatogenous retinal detachment.

Clinical Features

Ophthalmoscopically, lattice degeneration appears as one or more linear bands of retinal thinning located in the equatorial region. Fine white lines, which account for the name lattice degeneration (Fig. 8-8), are only present in about 10 percent of lesions. Pigmentary disturbances within the band of retinal thinning, however, are present in most cases (Fig. 8-9). Lattice degen-

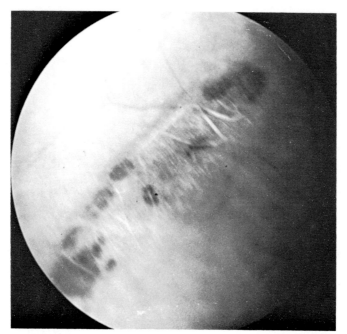

FIG. 8-8. Fundus photogr
of lattice degeneration of
retina, showing typical w
lines.

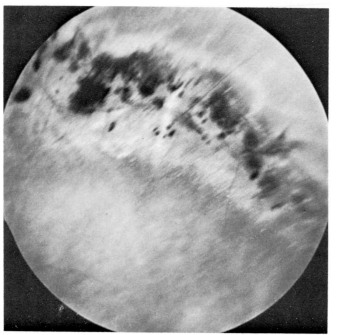

FIG. 8-9. Fundus photogr
of lattice degeneration,
showing pigmented area
retinal thinning but no w
lines.

eration is more common superiorly and is seen less frequently near the inferior equator. It is considerably less common in the horizontal meridians. In most cases, the lesions of lattice degeneration are arranged parallel to the ora serrata. Less commonly, the lesions are oriented obliquely or even perpendicular to the ora serrata.

In some patients retinal thinning and pigmentary disturbance are found along the retinal vessels. This condition is similar to typical lattice degeneration; it has been referred to as radial perivascular chorioretinal degeneration.[2]

Biomicroscopy of the vitreous adjacent to lattice degeneration may reveal rather typical changes. The vitreous gel is firmly attached to the margin of the lesion. There is usually a clear pocket of fluid vitreous over the central thin portion of each lesion.

Retinal holes can often be observed in lattice degeneration. Two types of holes have been recognized. Round or atrophic holes are usually found centrally within the thin portion of the lesion and are not usually associated with vitreous traction. Horseshoe-shaped holes occur most commonly on the posterior edge of the lesion and are associated with severe vitreous traction. In many cases, multiple holes of both types are present. These holes sometimes lead to retinal detachment.[11] The relationship of lattice degeneration to retinal detachment is considered in more detail later.

Pathology

Light microscopy of lattice degeneration reveals thinning and disorganization of the retina, with little or no alteration in the choroid (Fig. 8-10). The involved area frequently shows melanin-laden macrophages, which explains the pigmentation seen clinically. The blood vessels in the inner portion of the lesion are usually patent and there is often a fibrous tissue thickening of their walls (Fig. 8-11). These patent but thickened blood vessels correlate with the white lines seen clinically.

The adjacent vitreous also shows histopathologic alterations. Strands of condensed vitreous are present at the margin of the lesion, often causing the retinal tissue to be tented or elevated. There is a clear area over the center of the lesion; this corresponds to the pocket of liquid vitreous observed clinically (Fig. 8-10).

Pathogenesis

The pathogenesis of lattice degeneration is poorly understood. Whether it is purely an effect of the vitreous traction, or whether the retinal vessels play a primary role is difficult to ascertain. In contrast to the situation in paving stone degeneration, the choroidal vessels appear to play little if any role.

Relationship to Retinal Detachment and Candidates for Treatment

Lattice degeneration of the retina is present in about 6 percent of adult eyes. Since the incidence of retinal detachment is much lower, it is apparent that

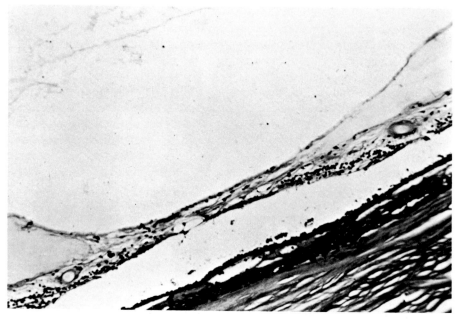

FIG. 8-10. Low-power photomicrograph of lattice degeneration. Note the retinal thinning, disorganization, and overlying pocket of fluid vitreous. (Courtesy of Dr. WR Green)

FIG. 8-11. Low-power photomicrograph of lattice degeneration, showing thickening of the retinal blood vessel wall in the involved area. (Courtesy of Dr. WR Green) (Hematoxylin-eosin stain; ×25)

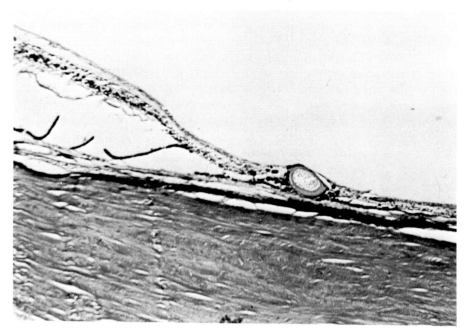

most cases of lattice degeneration will not progress to detachment and, therefore, do not need to be treated. Consequently, the clinician should attempt to recognize those cases which represent a greater likelihood of developing a retinal detachment.

There are certain factors which suggest that treatment should be considered. The first such factor is the presence of retinal holes. If there are no holes, treatment is rarely indicated. Treatment is also unnecessary when holes are present but asymptomatic and there is no subretinal fluid. Symptomatic holes with subretinal fluid should usually be treated. Another factor is the location of the lattice degeneration. One should be more inclined to treat areas near the superior or superotemporal equator, but less inclined to treat those located inferiorly.

The status of the opposite eye is an important consideration. A history of retinal detachment secondary to lattice degeneration in the opposite eye should lend support in favor of treatment. The age of the patient is another consideration. One is less inclined to treat lattice degeneration in an older or debilitated patient, and more inclined in a young person who has more years during which a retinal detachment could occur. Clearly, the need for treatment of this condition is quite controversial, and each case must be individually evaluated, with consideration given to the entire clinical situation.

Treatment

Lattice degeneration can be treated with cryotherapy, photocoagulation, or a scleral buckling procedure. Cryotherapy is effective in those cases with lesions in the periphery which can be reached by scleral depression. For lesions located more posteriorly, a small conjunctival incision will be necessary in order to reach the lesion. Light treatment to produce moderate pigmentation around the lesion will usually be sufficient.

Photocoagulation, using the xenon arc photocoagulator or the argon laser, is also an effective means for treating this condition. It should be reserved for more posteriorly located lesions in eyes which have relatively clear media. The lesion should be surrounded with photocoagulation burns, made with enough energy to create a surrounding chorioretinal adhesion.

A scleral buckling procedure should be used in cases of lattice degeneration which have progressed to retinal detachment. It can also be used if there is severe vitreous traction on the margin, with retinal holes and impending detachment. The exact technique will depend on the preference of the surgeon.

NONSPECIFIC PERIPHERAL CHORIORETINAL ATROPHY

In many patients, nonspecific diffuse pigmentary changes may be observed in the peripheral retina. These changes are not compatible with the characteristic findings of lattice or paving stone degeneration and are probably of little

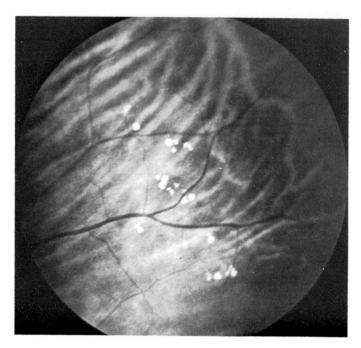

FIG. 8-12. Fundus photograph of scattered drusen in the fundus periphery.

clinical significance. They are more common in older patients and may be related to choroidal vascular disease. The pathogenesis may be similar to that of the atrophic senile macular degeneration commonly found in the posterior pole of older patients.

Peripheral drusen (Fig. 8-12; see also Fig. 3-11 in Chap. 3) are similar to the drusen seen in the posterior pole in senile macular degeneration. One type of drusen, however, known as an ora serrata pearl, is located at the ora serrata, often in a dentate process (see also in Chap. 1). It is found in 20 percent of autopsy eyes[5] and may be related to chronic traction of the zonules of the lens at the ora serrata. This may lead to proliferation of the retinal pigment epithelium, with laying down of basement membrane material in the form of drusen (Fig. 8-13).

PERIPHERAL EXUDATIVE HEMORRHAGIC CHORIORETINOPATHY (PEHCR)

This condition, also known as peripheral or eccentric disciform degeneration, or hemorrhagic detachment of the retinal pigment epithelium, has been recognized with increasing frequency in recent years.[8]

Clinical and Pathologic Features

PEHCR (Fig. 8-14) is characterized by a peripheral fundus mass associated with hemorrhage, exudates, and, frequently, a serous retinal detachment. It

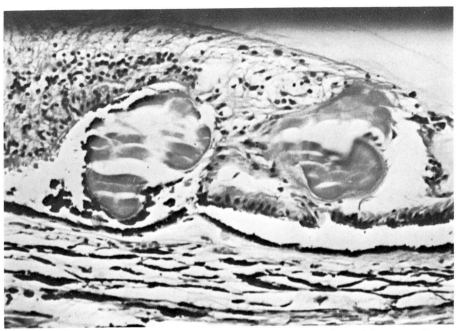

FIG. 8-13. Photomicrograph of oral serrata pearls, i.e., calcified drusen at the ora serrata. (AFIP accession no. 1326686) (Hematoxylin-eosin stain; ×250)

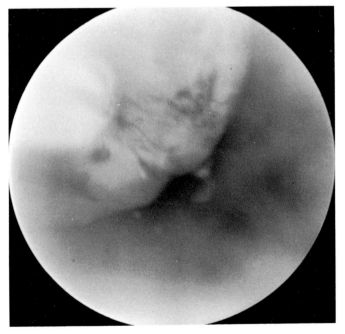

FIG. 8-14. Peripheral fundus mass secondary to peripheral exudative hemorrhagic chorioretinopathy (PEHCR).

may vary from dark to reddish pink, depending on the amount of hemorrhage or vascularity within the lesion. Recent clinical and pathologic studies have suggested that this condition occurs secondary to neovascularization that grows from the choroid through defects in Bruch's membrane into the space beneath the retinal pigment epithelium. These abnormal vessels lead to exudation and recurrent hemorrhages, finally culminating in a fibrous disciform scar. New blood vessels within the lesion and on its surface may grow into the vitreous and produce extensive hemorrhage. PEHCR is often associated with other changes, such as drusen and macular degeneration.

Although few cases have been studied pathologically, PEHCR appears to be identical to senile disciform degeneration which is seen in the posterior pole.

Differential Diagnosis

In some cases it may be extremely difficult to differentiate PEHCR from a malignant melanoma of the peripheral choroid. The degree of hemorrhage and exudation is usually greater than one would expect with a melanoma of comparable size. Vitreous hemorrhage commonly occurs with PEHCR, but is relatively rare with small peripheral melanomas. Fluorescein angiography may be helpful in some cases by demonstrating the subretinal neovascular membrane and hypofluorescence corresponding to the hemorrhage. These are features not usually seen with choroidal melanoma. In difficult cases the ^{32}P test can be used. It is usually negative, or the uptake is much less than with a melanoma of comparable size.[7]

PEHCR may also resemble a capillary hemangioma of the retina as seen in von Hippel-Lindau disease (see Chap. 7). Even though PEHCR causes hemorrhages, exudates, and subretinal fluid, it lacks the typical dilated feeder vessels associated with capillary hemangioma. The family history is negative, whereas von Hippel-Lindau disease is usually transmitted in an autosomal dominant pattern.

Some confusion also exists as to the relationship between PEHCR and the adult form of Coats' disease (see in Chap. 6). The latter has often been used as a "wastebasket" diagnosis, and probably incorporates a number of entities such as the intraretinal macroaneurysm seen in hypertensive patients and intraocular inflammations of any cause. It is likely that many cases of adult Coats' disease are actually examples of PEHCR.

Treatment

Most cases of PEHCR do not require treatment. If the exudation and subretinal fluid are progressing posteriorly towards the macula, delimiting cryotherapy or photocoagulation will have only partial success. If vitreous hemorrhage occurs and does not resolve sufficiently in 6 months, vitrectomy might be considered. No medications are known to be helpful.

REFERENCES

1. **Foos RY:** Senile retinoschisis. Relationship to cystoid degeneration. Trans Am Acad Ophthalmol Otolaryngol 74:33–51, 1970

2. **Hagler WS, Crosswell HH:** Radial perivascular chorioretinal degeneration and retinal detachment. Trans Am Acad Ophthalmol Otolaryngol 72:203–216, 1968

3. **Hagler WS, Woldoff HS:** Retinal detachment in relation to senile retinoschisis. Trans Am Acad Ophthalmol Otolaryngol 77:99–113, 1973

4. **Johnson BL:** Proteinaceous cysts of the ciliary epithelium. II. Their occurrence in non-myelomatous hypergammaglobulinemic conditions. Arch Ophthalmol 84:171–175, 1970

5. **Lonn LI, Smith TR:** Ora serrata pearls. Arch Ophthalmol 77:809–813, 1967

6. **O'Malley P, Allen RA, Straatsma BR, O'Malley CC:** Paving stone degeneration of the retina. Arch Ophthalmol 73:169–182, 1965

7. **Shields JA:** Accuracy and limitation of the ^{32}P test in the diagnosis of ocular tumors. An analysis of 500 cases. Ophthalmology 85:950–966, 1978

8. **Silva VB, Brockhurst RJ:** Hemorrhagic detachment of the peripheral retinal pigment epithelium. Arch Ophthalmol 94:1295–1300, 1976

9. **Straatsma BR, Foos RY:** Typical and reticular degenerative retinoschisis. Am J Ophthalmol 75:551–575, 1973

10. **Straatsma BR, Zeegan PD, Foos, RY, Feman SS, Shabo AL:** Lattice degeneration of the retina. XXX Edward Jackson Memorial Lecture. Am J Ophthalmol 77:619–649, 1974

11. **Tillery WV, Lucier AC:** Round atrophic holes in lattice degeneration—an important cause of phakic retinal detachment. Trans Am Acad Ophthalmol Otolaryngol 81:509–518, 1976

9

Retinal and Choroidal Detachment

Gonin[17, 18]first recognized the retinal break, or tear, as the etiology of retinal detachment. Since then, refinements in examination of the peripheral fundus have led to improved cure rates with surgery of this once almost universally blinding condition. Retinal detachment due to one or more retinal breaks is called rhegmatogenous detachment. It is characterized by serous elevation of the sensory retina due to an accumulation of fluid between the photoreceptor elements and the retinal pigment epithelium. The retinal break (or breaks) causing the detachment may be defined as a discontinuity in the sensory retina. To effect a cure, it is necessary to seal each of the retinal breaks which are present. Failure to close any break successfully will lead to continued detachment or redetachment of the retina.

Rhegmatogenous retinal detachment must be differentiated from secondary detachments. These occur most commonly as a result of tumors, intraocular inflammation, or pigment epithelial detachments, or from uveal effusion, as described by Schepens, Brockhurst, and Lam, in which no retinal break is usually present.[2, 26]

RETINAL BREAKS

Types of Retinal Breaks

Since the hallmark of a rhegmatogenous retinal detachment is the presence of retinal breaks, some discussion of the different types of retinal breaks is warranted. Common usage has led to the descriptive naming of some breaks as

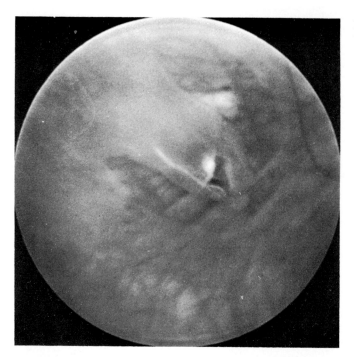

FIG. 9-1. Horseshoe tear of the retina.

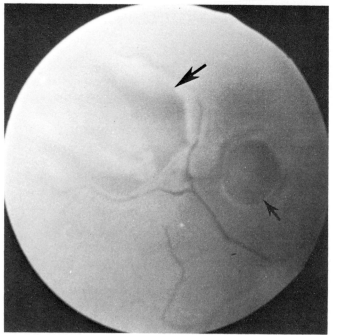

FIG. 9-2. Horseshoe tear within the fork of a retinal vessel *(large arrow)*. Posterior to the horseshoe is a round tear *(small arrow)* which has a free-floating operculum. Round breaks tend to be located more posteriorly than horseshoe breaks, which are delimited anteriorly by the posterior border of the vitreous base.

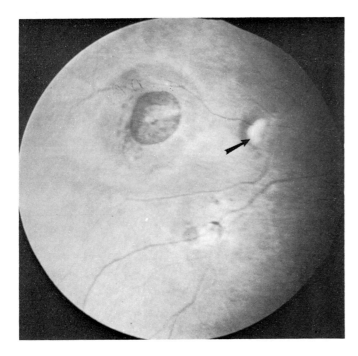

FIG. 9-3. Round retinal break with a free-floating operculum (*arrow*). A small rim of subretinal fluid surrounds the break.

horseshoe or flap tears (Figs. 9-1 and 9-2), and of others as operculated tears, in which a plug of retina has been pulled free and floats in the vitreous cavity like a small manhole cover (Fig. 9-3). Other retinal breaks may be round or oval atrophic areas.

Retinal breaks may be associated with degenerative conditions of the retina, such as lattice degeneration (Fig. 9-4, Plate 3, *B*). Some reports indicate that in as many as 30 percent of all detachments the retinal breaks are associated with areas of lattice degeneration.[10, 31, 32] Byer, however, monitored 204 untreated patients with lattice degeneration and forecasted only a 0.3 percent incidence of detachment.[4] Breaks in lattice degeneration may have the appearance of a horseshoe tear which occurs either at the edge or along the posterior border of the lattice, or may be round small holes within the lattice degeneration itself (Fig. 9-5). If a large area of lattice degeneration is present and a tear occurs on the weakened posterior edge of the lattice, much as one would tear the serrations of a postage stamp, a giant tear greater than 90 degrees may develop (Plate 3, *C*).

Another type of tear is the retinal dialysis which so often follows blunt trauma. This type of tear is likely to start as several oval breaks along the posterior border of the vitreous base. The breaks then become confluent to form the typical crescent-shaped dialysis. Some controversy exists as to whether or not all of these dialyses are traumatic and, particularly, whether some that are located in the inferior temporal quadrants are actually congenital. This is discussed in greater detail later in the chapter, under Traumatic Retinal Detachment.

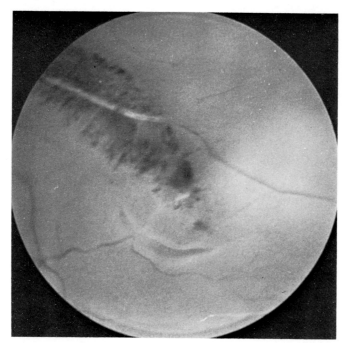

FIG. 9-4. Retinal break at edge of an area of lattice degeneration, causing reti detachment.

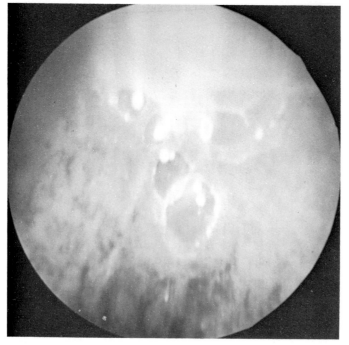

FIG. 9-5. Multiple round retinal breaks within latt degeneration.

Posterior Vitreous Detachment

Retinal break formation frequently occurs at the time of a posterior vitreous detachment (PVD), a condition which increases in incidence with age. Two types of PVD may occur, a symptomatic one and a milder asymptomatic variety.

A symptomatic PVD is usually described by the patient as being preceded by flashes of light, which are often worse in the dark, and then by the onset of what appears to be a cobweb, fly, or thread in the field of vision. If a mild vitreous hemorrhage occurs at the time of the PVD, the patient may also mention the presence of dust or soot in his vision. If the hemorrhage is severe the patient's vision may suddenly become completely obscured. An asymptomatic posterior vitreous detachment is much less apt to cause a retinal break than a symptomatic one, but all cases demand a careful examination of the fundus periphery to rule out a retinal break. The cobweb floater appears to the ophthalmologist as an annular opacity (Fig. 9-6). In addition, slit lamp biomicroscopy may reveal the collapsed vitreous gel (Fig. 9-7).

Some years ago Stratford and Shafer[33] described an extremely important clinical finding, the presence of pigment dust in the vitreous gel behind the lens in phakic patients with acute posterior vitreous detachment, and recognized that this was virtually a pathognomonic sign of retinal break or retinal detachment (Fig. 9-8). The same does not hold true for aphakic patients, however, who often have pigment dust in the vitreous but no retinal break.

FIG. 9-6. Annular opacity (*arrow*) in the midvitreous following a posterior vitreous detachment. (Courtesy of Armed Forces Institute of Pathology)

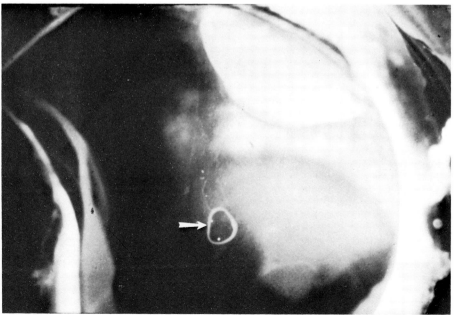

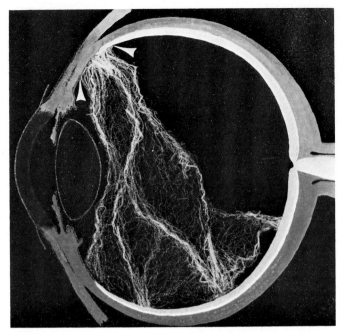

FIG. 9-7. Posterior vitreou detachment: Collapsed vitreous gel with opticall empty space posteriorly. vitreous base (*arrows*) remains attached to the peripheral retina and straddles the ora serrata.

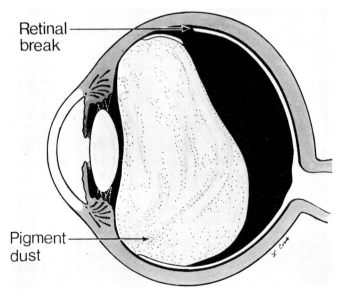

Retinal break

Pigment dust

FIG. 9-8. Posterior vitreo detachment in a phakic e Note the pigment dust present in the vitreous ge In phakic eyes, this is aln a pathognomonic sign of retinal break formation o retinal detachment.

When severe hemorrhage has occurred, it is difficult for the ophthalmologist to examine the fundus, and prompt hospitalization of the patient, with complete bed rest, is indicated. Binocular patches should be applied, and the patient's head should be elevated to allow settling of the blood in the retrohyaloid space. One must assume that a retinal break is present until proved otherwise, unless the physician knows that he is dealing with a diabetic who has had vitreous hemorrhages before.

In most cases, the retinal break will be above the horizontal raphe, but this is certainly not an absolute rule and the patient must be monitored carefully until the ora serrata can be examined throughout 360 degrees.

Pathogenesis of Retinal Breaks

Although vitreoretinal traction is a major factor in the development of retinal breaks, other factors may also play a role. Zonular traction tufts, described by Foos,[11] are drawn from the surrounding retinal surface towards the ciliary body at an acute angle. Several attached zonules can usually be seen at or immediately behind the tip of the tuft. The retina at the base of the tufts shows varying degrees of trophic change, including cystic degeneration and thinning. Tractional alterations are manifested by elevation of the retina at the base, which is either rounded and somewhat cystic, has raised margins and a depressed center, or shows slightly elevated folds radiating posteriorly from the center of the base. The underlying pigment epithelium is often darkened, and occasionally one can observe dispersion of pigment clumps into the retina at the base of the tuft.

Zonular traction tufts of the peripheral retina were present in 9 percent of 1500 autopsy eyes examined by Foos.[11] The lesions were present at birth and in 81 percent of the cases were in the nasal quadrants. Full-thickness holes in the base of the tufts were present in 4 percent of the cases and partial-thickness holes were found in 10 percent.

Many retinal breaks occur in association with vitreous hemorrhage, supporting the clinical impression that vitreoretinal traction is more marked over retinal vessels. Spencer and Foos have noted apparent paravascular vitreoretinal attachments,[29, 30] which may be why tears commonly involve retinal blood vessels.

In a later study Foos pointed out that the cause of surface breaks probably is a multifactorial series of events.[12] Thinning of the internal limiting lamina may take place during development. A subsurface retinal degeneration may be complicated by vitreous incarceration or epiretinal membrane formation. During PVD any of these factors can cause peeling of the retinal surface and, ultimately, large surface breaks.

Incidence of Retinal Breaks after Posterior Vitreous Detachment

Jaffe,[20] Linder,[23] and Tasman[35] have each studied a series of patients with symptomatic PVD; the incidence of retinal breaks occurring in these series ranged from 10 to 15 percent. In addition, Linder found in his series that when retinal breaks occurred with PVD, all were above the horizontal meridian. This is in contrast to the work of Jaffe and of Tasman, who found that 85 percent and 65 percent, respectively, of the tears occurred above the horizontal meridian. However, all three authors reported that about 5 percent of patients in their series sustained vitreous hemorrhage without retinal break formation when symptomatic PVD occurred. This is a significant figure to remember and, as indicated earlier, most likely the vitreous hemorrhage occurs because of traction on a retinal blood vessel. In addition, patients who have a symptomatic PVD and who demonstrate small hemorrhages along the posterior border of the vitreous base bear careful watching during the first month after the onset of symptoms, since a certain number of these patients will develop retinal breaks within this time.

Treatment of Retinal Breaks

The clinician must decide which patients with retinal break formation will require prophylactic treatment, and what type of treatment is indicated. The series of Colyear and Pischel[7] in 1956 and the later work of Davis[10] demonstrate that symptomatic horseshoe tears have a greater than 50 percent chance of leading to retinal detachment. Thus, there seems to be little question that such tears should be treated prophylactically. If there is a patent retinal vessel in the flap of the horseshoe tear, or bridging the mouth of the tear, we favor a localized scleral buckling procedure, with diathermy to close the retinal vessel. If these patients are treated merely with cryotherapy, vitreous hemorrhage may recur at a later date because the unsupported retinal vessel has not been occluded. If there is no vessel problem but merely subretinal fluid beneath the edges of the tear, then a localized scleral buckling technique, using either cryotherapy and a silicone sponge or diathermy and a bed, seems adequate. When the horseshoe tear is completely flat and there is no vessel problem, simple cryotherapy, applied transconjunctivally, proves to be a satisfactory means of management.

The operculated tear (in which a small operculum of retina is floating freely in the vitreous cavity) is less dangerous than a horseshoe tear. Operculated tears have only about a 16 percent chance of detachment.[2, 7] These breaks respond well to cryotherapy. If the tear is too posterior to reach with the cryoprobe, it may be treated with laser photocoagulation, provided there has been no vitreous hemorrhage. When there has been a significant amount of vitreous hemorrhage it is better to treat such breaks with cryotherapy, even if it means making an incision in the conjunctiva to avoid passing heat through the vitreous cavity.

Atrophic retinal breaks, which are most often asymptomatic, can usually be safely observed. Again, from the work of Davis[10] and of Byer,[3, 5, 6] it is known that such breaks have a less than 10 percent chance of causing a retinal detachment. Moreover, 7 to 8 percent of the population have undetected retinal breaks. It may therefore be concluded from the fact that the incidence of retinal detachment is only 0.01 percent that most atrophic retinal breaks will not lead to a detached retina and therefore require no treatment.[24]

A retinal dialysis can usually be closed successfully with cryotherapy and probably should be treated even though it may be in the inferior temporal quadrant, because a detachment that occurs secondary to the dialysis progresses slowly before becoming symptomatic when it finally reaches the macula.

Giant tears of the retina (Plate 3, C) require very specialized care, and their management is continually undergoing change. Freeman[13] has described the use, in the past, of intravitreal balloons to help unfold the inverted flaps, then of operating tables on which the patient can be turned upside down so that air may be injected beneath the flap, and, more recently, of vitrectomy to try to remove the diseased vitreous at the time of retinal repair. Despite all of these heroic measures, the overall results with giant tears are less satisfactory than one would desire, and there are continued efforts to find improved techniques to combat this devastating form of retinal detachment. Still, one must attempt to treat these cases since Freeman has shown a high incidence of retinal break formation in the fellow eye of giant tear patients.[14]

RHEGMATOGENOUS RETINAL DETACHMENT

Patients with rhegmatogenous retinal detachment may be divided into those who are phakic and those who are aphakic. Aphakic patients who develop retinal detachment may be treated in the same way as those in whom the lens has not been removed. Both groups have a good surgical prognosis for reattachment.

The age of peak incidence of retinal detachment in phakic patients is 50 to 60 years in males and 60 to 70 years in females. Phakic patients with retinal detachments predominate by approximately a three to one count, but aphakic patients actually have a much higher incidence of retinal detachment in that approximately 2 percent of patients who are aphakic can be expected to develop a retinal detachment, even when the prior cataract extraction has been uncomplicated. The increased incidence of retinal detachment in aphakia may be due to the prevalence of intracapsular lens extractions: with this procedure, the vitreous gel is no longer supported by the lens and often prolapses into the anterior chamber, placing traction on the posterior border of the vitreous base.

Patients with aphakic detachments often have very small breaks in the region of the ora serrata that may be extremely hard to detect. With identification of the retinal breaks, however, their prognosis is good, although most reports show a slightly lower reattachment rate than for the phakic group.[1]

With the increased popularity of extracapsular techniques such as phacoemulsification, the problem of treating aphakic detachment has changed somewhat. Shafer[28] found no difference in the aphakic detachment after phacoemulsification and after intracapsular extraction. Sometimes, however, the retinal break may be hard to find because of the ring of capsule which is so often left at the pupillary border. When phacoemulsification was first used, one of the publicized assets of the procedure was that the posterior capsule was left intact, on the theory that the incidence of aphakic retinal detachment might be reduced. However, a year or two after the procedure many patients began to develop thickening of the posterior capsule and required a secondary procedure to incise the posterior membrane. Because of this many surgeons now remove the posterior capsule at the time of phacoemulsification.

One cannot overemphasize the hazards that accompany phacoemulsification. When it is uncomplicated it certainly leaves a very desirable result in that the patient is back to fairly normal activity in a short period of time and may be fitted with a contact lens much sooner than after a conventional intracapsular cataract extraction. On the other hand, if complications do occur during surgery they are much more difficult to manage. Such complications include loss of vitreous and dislocation of the lens or its nucleus into the vitreous cavity.

The importance of examining the fellow eye of patients with aphakic retinal detachment is well documented in a series of 185 patients with unilateral aphakic retinal detachment.[1] In that study the authors determined that the frequency of later retinal detachment in aphakic fellow eyes was 26 percent. This was almost four times higher than the 7 percent frequency rate for phakic eyes. Despite the high incidence of detachment 94 percent of the aphakic group had a final visual acuity of 20/60 or better in the second eye. This was undoubtedly due to the fact that the macula was still attached in 57 percent of the second eyes compared to only 17 percent of the first eyes. Because of the high incidence of bilateral retinal detachment in aphakic eyes, prophylactic therapy of breaks in such eyes is usually indicated.

History of Scleral Buckling

Present-day success in the repair of retinal detachment is due in large part to Schepens and Custodis, both of whom contributed significantly to the scleral buckling techniques which are presently used. In the 1950s, Schepens[27] popularized the encircling buckling procedure, using first a polyethylene encircling tube and later, at the suggestion of P. R. McDonald, silicone rubber. The use of silicone rubber implants in association with encircling silicone rubber bands is now well accepted.

The credit for scleral buckling goes to Custodis[9] who developed the polyvinyl alcohol (Polyviol) explant, which was sewn over the retinal break, and popularized the fact that it was not necessary to drain subretinal fluid if the buckle could be properly placed beneath the retinal breaks. Later, Lincoff and colleagues[22] developed silicone rubber sponges, which were better tolerated by the eye and, with the advent of cryotherapy, led to repopularization of Custodis' theory of explants without subretinal fluid drainage.

Drainage of Subretinal Fluid

The attempt to avoid subretinal fluid drainage during surgery is due of course to the fact that this is the riskiest part of the operation. However, certain precautions can be taken to minimize the risks. Probably first and foremost is the proper location of the site of drainage. One wishes to drain where the retina is definitely elevated and preferably where there are no choroidal vessels. Ideal sites for subretinal fluid drainage are either just above or just below the horizontal rectus muscles if subretinal fluid is located in these areas. It is important, as Freeman et al.[15, 16] have stressed, to transilluminate the sclera before beginning a site for drainage of subretinal fluid in order to be sure that one has selected an area where choroidal vessels are not present. Application of diathermy to the lips of the scleral cutdown and to the choroid itself are additional factors which may help to minimize hemorrhage. When a perforation is made for drainage of subretinal fluid the surgeon should make sure that his assistants have released traction on the eye so that drainage is not performed while the intraocular pressure is elevated, thereby lessening the chance for retinal incarceration. The fluid should be allowed to flow smoothly without undue pressure on the eye since again this might lead to incarceration of the retina.

Ideally, if one can close the retinal break with the scleral buckle and not occlude the central retinal artery at the same time, one may elect to not drain subretinal fluid. Often the retina will be reattached within 24 to 48 hours following surgery.

The patients in whom explants are used, and who still require drainage of subretinal fluid, include those in whom the retinal break cannot be successfully closed or at least approximated to the buckle; those with very thin sclera, since the surgeon must be concerned about pulling out of the sutures if the eye is not softened prior to tying them up; and those with glaucoma, since, again, tightening the sutures would create excess tension, which would threaten to occlude the central retinal artery.

DISORDERS ASSOCIATED WITH RETINAL DETACHMENT

CHOROIDAL COLOBOMA

Certain conditions, both congenital and hereditary, may be associated with rhegmatogenous retinal detachment. One of these is congenital coloboma of the choroid (Fig. 9-9). Retinal detachment, a real hazard to colobomatous eyes, was observed in 10 of 24 eyes in Jesberg and Schepens' series.[21] They noted two types of retinal detachment associated with choroidal coloboma. The first type included cases in which the coloboma was no more than an incidental finding. Obvious retinal breaks were found, apparently unrelated to the coloboma, and their closure resulted in reattachment of the retina.

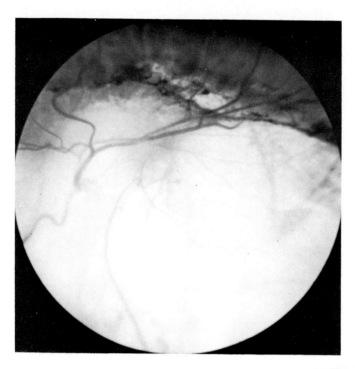

FIG. 9-9. Large coloboma
the optic nerve, retina, ar
choroid located inferiorly
Retinal breaks tend to oc
along the margin of the
coloboma and, when loca
within the diaphanous
membrane overlying the
coloboma, are virtually
impossible to identify.

The second type of retinal detachment which they observed appeared
to be definitely related to the choroidal coloboma and either was inferotemporal, with demarcation lines, or was total. It was fairly smooth, with
high retinal folds or large balloons. In these cases they believed that the retinal
detachment was due to one or more breaks located in the colobomatous area.
Such breaks are extremely hard to detect because of the lack of contrast
afforded by the white scleral background and the diaphanous nature of the
overlying retinal membrane. In addition, it is possible that a break in
the membrane might occur in an area of the coloboma which was hidden
behind the scleral edge of the posterior staphyloma, or in the region of the
greatly distorted inferior ora serrata. The presence of such a break may be
signified by the presence of a recent hemorrhage in the colobomatous area;
this sign must be given due consideration when present. The edges of the
colobomatous area must be carefully examined by stereoscopic ophthalmoscopy for indications of elevation connected with the retinal detachment. It has
been found that diagnosis can be helped by the use of a slit lamp and flat
corneal contact lens as well as by the binocular indirect ophthalmoscope.

Colobomatous eyes respond poorly to surgery and are frequently difficult to work on technically because they are often microphthalmic. Surgical
diathermy designed to delimit the coloboma may effect a cure in certain
patients. Such diathermy should be applied with utmost care, using a small
diathermy electrode. This procedure is preferable to cryotherapy since accurate minimal applications are essential when treatments are applied along the

edge of the coloboma, because all nerve fibers peripheral to an application are sacrificed. When a coloboma involving the disc is encountered, one cannot treat the entire extent of the defect without interfering with the nerve fibers from all quadrants. Occasionally, however, treatment limited to only the elevated portion of the coloboma's edge may be attempted. It is obvious that the adhesive chorioretinitis which is caused by diathermy cannot be produced when choroid and retina are either extremely atrophic or absent. Thus, treatment in the colobomatous area would probably be of no value in closing retinal breaks that might be present over the coloboma.

Retinal breaks away from the coloboma should be treated first since every application of the diathermy along the edge of the coloboma in the proximity of the disc causes loss of function of the related nerve fibers from peripheral areas.

GIANT RETINAL BREAK WITH COLOBOMA OF THE LENS AND ZONULES

Hovland, Schepens, and Freeman[19] have described eight cases of bilateral retinal detachment with giant retinal breaks associated with a nasal coloboma of the lens and zonule. These ocular defects were observed in young children who had other systemic abnormalities.

The salient ocular features were the bilateral defects in the lens, zonule, and retina. The lenticular defect was a nasal coloboma which appeared as an equatorial flattening of the lens. The zonule was absent nasally over an arc of 90 to 135 degrees in most eyes. The retinas had giant breaks which extended from 90 to 360 degrees and involved the nasal quadrants in 12 of 13 eyes having a giant break. Additionally, four eyes showed a large retinal hole with rolled edges located posterior to the giant break. No obvious abnormalities were noted in the vitreous nor were any of the ciliary processes pulled centrally. The surgical and visual prognosis in such eyes is poor: of the 16 eyes in this series, only 4 had the retina successfully reattached, and of these, only one had better than light-perception vision.

EHLERS-DANLOS SYNDROME

An association between familial retinal detachment and Ehlers-Danlos syndrome has been described. Retinal breaks in affected patients do not seem to have a uniformly characteristic appearance. All the retinal breaks in a series reported by Pemberton et al.[25] were located temporally and were accompanied by evidence of strong vitreous traction, such as rolled edges, areas that were white in the absence of pressure, and horseshoe tears with visible adherent vitreous membranes. Premature degeneration and collapse of the vitreous body occurred in all the eyes.

Many associated ocular findings are present in the Ehlers-Danlos syndrome, such as epicanthus, ptosis, and hypotony of the extrinsic muscles, often resulting in strabismus. Laxity of the palpebral tissues is evidenced by the presence of Metenier's sign, an unusual ease in everting the upper eyelid. Blue sclera and myopia have also been frequently noted. Keratoconus, ectopia of the lens, postoperative dehiscence of cataract wounds, and bilateral corneal lacerations as a result of minor trauma have also been observed. Additional ophthalmoscopic findings have included angioid streaks, equatorial pigmentary changes, and macular degeneration. Vitreous hemorrhage has also been described in patients with this syndrome.

The Ehlers-Danlos syndrome is an autosomal-dominant inherited disorder of connective tissue which is manifested clinically by hyperelastic, fragile skin and hyperlaxity of the joints. Wounds of the skin have a tendency to gape, and poor healing and scarring are common. Although present at birth, the signs of Ehlers-Danlos syndrome usually become manifest when the child begins to walk. The most striking example of joint hyperextensibility is noted in the hands, particularly in the thumbs and fingers. Some patients can extend these digits so that they touch the wrist.

There are several important considerations in the clinical management of retinal detachment in patients having this connective tissue syndrome. For example, there is a definite tendency for vitreous hemorrhage to occur, so that it is advisable to decrease the intensity of diathermy or cryotherapy applications. Because of the frequency and prominence of traction-producing vitreous membranes, a scleral buckling procedure is indicated when possible. If the sclera is quite thin, photocoagulation or cryosurgery is preferable to the use of diathermy. Relatively innocuous areas of retinal disease in fellow eyes have been known to develop retinal breaks quite rapidly. For this reason, follow-up examinations of the fellow eye should be frequent and detailed.

MARFAN'S SYNDROME

Another systemic condition frequently associated with retinal detachment is Marfan's syndrome. Marfan's patients are characterized by arachnodactyly (elongation of long bones) and autosomal dominant inheritance. In patients with this syndrome, retinal breaks are usually located in the equatorial region. Often the pupil fails to dilate well, and since the lens is frequently subluxated, ophthalmoscopy is difficult and breaks may be easily missed. With subluxation of the lens, part of the pupil is phakic and part is aphakic (Fig. 9-10). By tilting the patient's head appropriately, one can sometimes move the lens so that the entire pupil becomes phakic or aphakic, resulting in an improvement of the fundus image. Tilting up the ophthalmoscope mirror and using high-powered condensing lenses such as a +30-diopter (30D) lens will also improve ophthalmoscopy.

Lens removal should be performed only as a last resort, and one should expect vitreous loss during lens extraction and therefore should be prepared to handle this complication when it occurs. If the lens is dislocated but clear, and if retinal breaks can be identified, the patient may be managed in a conventional fashion by a standard buckling procedure. However, individuals with Marfan's syndrome may develop open-angle glaucoma postoperatively because of angle abnormalities related to the syndrome itself.

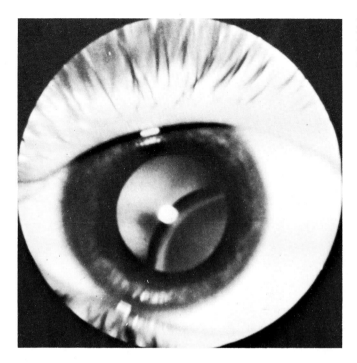

FIG. 9-10. Subluxated lens in Marfan's syndrome. Part of the pupil is phakic and the other part aphakic.

BLUNT TRAUMA

Another etiology of retinal detachment, and a significant one, especially among youngsters, is trauma. The fact that trauma is the most common cause of juvenile retinal detachment helps to explain the greater incidence of this condition in males than in females.

Blunt trauma and penetrating injuries both can cause detachment. However, in the case of blunt trauma there may be a latent period of several months or even years between the injury and a diagnosis of detachment. This is understandable for two reasons: firstly, children are often reluctant to report an injury or symptom, and secondly, many traumatic detachments start inferiorly and do not cause a subjective awareness until the macula is threatened.

Characteristics of Traumatic Detachments

Because traumatic retinal detachments may be asymptomatic initially, one or more demarcation lines are often present (Fig. 9-11) and, when found, confirm a duration of several months. A multiplicity of demarcation lines indicates successive increases in the size of the detachment and is evidence that chorioretinal adhesions cannot be counted on to wall off the elevated retina. The detachments are seldom bullous, but tend instead to be smooth and flat (Fig. 9-12). Fixed retinal folds are rare, although they may occur, and intraretinal cysts may be present if the detachment is old. These disappear spontaneously, usually within a few days, if the retina reattaches after surgery.

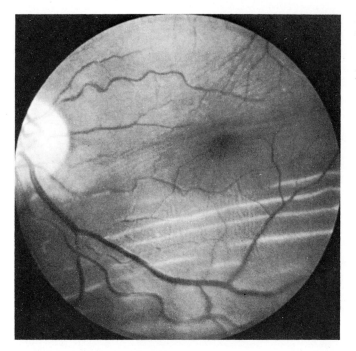

FIG. 9-11. Multiple demarcation lines in a long-standing traumatic retinal detachment which just invaded the macula.

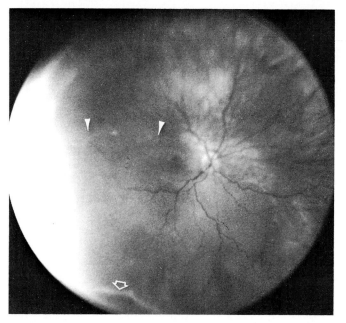

FIG. 9-12. Equator-plus photograph of retinal detachment with inferior temporal traumatic dialys (hollow arrow). The marg of the detachment is indicated by the solid arro

Traumatic Retinal Dialysis

Typically, the retinal break seen after blunt trauma begins, as mentioned earlier in this chapter, as a tear along the posterior border of the vitreous base. Gradually the break takes on the classic crescentic configuration of a dialysis. Less common is a radial break, which may occur acutely after blunt trauma (Fig. 9-13).

Dialyses tend to occur primarily in the inferotemporal and the superior nasal quadrants. Cox, Schepens, and Freeman[8] noted that traumatic dialyses occur most often superonasally, but in our experience we have seen more inferior temporal than superior nasal traumatic dialyses. Of course, any of the quadrants and sometimes more than one may be the site of a dialysis, so that careful searching of the ora serrata for 360 degrees is imperative (Plate 3, *D*).

When the retina tears along both the anterior and the posterior borders of the vitreous base, the vitreous base itself may become avulsed, at which time it may hang like a pigmented loop in the vitreous cavity, dangling from its underlying strip of attached retina and pigment epithelium (Fig. 9-14). When avulsion of the vitreous base is present superonasally or inferotemporally, it is considered pathognomonic of traumatic retinal detachment.

The question arises as to whether traumatic dialyses occur at the time of trauma or later. Weidenthal and Schepens[38] have shown, using pig eyes, how dialyses may occur at the time of contusion. In a prospective series begun in 1969, Tasman[36] followed up 52 eyes referred because of blunt trauma. Some 13 dialyses were noted in 10 patients in this group, and in all but one case the diagnosis was made within the first 3 weeks after injury. The one delay in diagnosis was due to the fact that vitreous hemorrhage obscured the ora serrata. It appears, therefore, that many dialyses do occur at the time of injury, although the possibility that later vitreoretinal changes will lead to dialysis is also likely. Thus, the importance of carefully examining the fundus periphery following blunt trauma, and of making sure that the ora has been visualized for 360 degrees, cannot be overemphasized.

Another controversial point is the question as to whether or not some inferotemporal dialyses represent congenital defects or are due to forgotten trauma. Winslow and Tasman[39] reviewed 176 patients with retinal detachment, some of whom had inferotemporal dialyses that were not related historically to any trauma. In addition, there were no objective signs of trauma. Of interest, however, was the fact that five superonasal dialyses were detected in this group of 176 patients and here, too, there were no objective signs of previous trauma and no history of trauma. Ideally, it would seem desirable to examine newborn infants to see whether or not inferotemporal congenital dialyses do in fact occur, but this still would not rule out the possibility of dialysis secondary to the trauma of birth, either from forceps or from contusion sustained while going through the birth canal. Such trauma might explain the bilateral inferior temporal dialyses which are occasionally seen.

One cannot negate the existence, however, of congenital inferior temporal dialyses, since Verdaguer et al. in Chile have described the pedigree of a family with this condition, which showed autosomal recessive inheritance.[37]

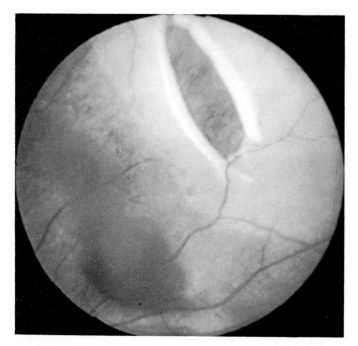

FIG. 9-13. Radial retinal break in a patient who sustained blunt trauma to eye.

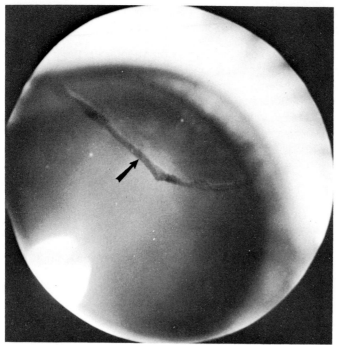

FIG. 9-14. Avulsed vitreo base *(arrow)* following blu trauma to the globe.

Detachment of the Ora Serrata with Pars Plana Breaks

Another form of traumatic peripheral retinal damage is extensive detachment of the ora serrata with retinal breaks in the nonpigmented epithelium of the pars plana ciliaris along the anterior border of the vitreous base. Pars plana breaks appear as small or large dialyses and usually cannot be seen without scleral depression. Although the epithelium of the pars plana ciliaris is thin and may appear more translucent than the posterior retina, this difference in thickness may not be striking enough to identify the detached ora serrata. The position of the ora, however, may be made more obvious by a variable amount of pigmentation which has been dragged from the underlying pigment epithelium. Another clue to the position of the ora is the presence of cystoid degeneration, which differentiates the extreme periphery of the retina from the epithelium of the pars plana. The contrast between thicker retina and thin pars plana is more marked in the folds of the often tented ora serrata, so that light reflected from the uveal blood vessels transmits as a reddish color through these tented areas, which can easily be mistaken for triangular breaks.

Direct Trauma to the Sclera

Direct trauma to the sclera or anterior to the equator can lead to choroidal rupture and hemorrhage, which is fairly characteristic in appearance. Such injuries are usually the result of a high-velocity missile, such as a BB or a foreign body shot out from under a rotary lawnmower, which contuses the globe but does not actually penetrate it. Examination of the ocular fundi reveals large irregular areas of choroidal dehiscence associated with hemorrhage, but interestingly enough there is frequently no evidence of a retinal break or dialysis. Such patients need merely to be watched; as they convalesce, pigmentary changes will be noted to occur in the affected area, leading to a chorioretinal scar. Occasionally, too, following blunt trauma, hemorrhage along the posterior border of the vitreous base can lead to a pigmentary chorioretinal scar suggestive of previous injury.

The type of direct contusion herein described differs from the choroidal rupture which occurs in the posterior pole as the result of an indirect shock wave from a blunt injury to the front of the eye. When an eye is contused, a force is transmitted through the ocular media to the back of the eye. Since Bruch's membrane is more elastic than the harder scleral shell, a dehiscence occurs within this layer, leading to the typical crescentic choroidal rupture so often present in the posterior pole, concentric with the disc (Fig. 9-15). If the rupture is not directly in the fovea, some improvement in vision may occur within the first 6 weeks after injury as the associated retinal hemorrhage clears. These lesions, however, in certain rare instances may later lead to subretinal neovascularization which, if far enough away from the fovea, may be amenable to argon laser photocoagulation.

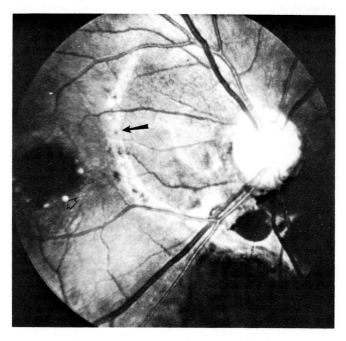

FIG. 9-15. Typical cresc
choroidal rupture *(solid
arrow)* that developed
between the disc and m
following blunt trauma.
addition, a macular hol
present which is
characterized by exudat
(hollow arrow) rimming
hole. The presence of su
exudates helps to estab}
the diagnosis of a
through-and-through
retinal break in the mac

CHOROIDAL DETACHMENT

Detachment Following Ocular Surgery

Choroidal detachment may occasionally be confused with retinal detachment. Most commonly this happens after a tension-lowering procedure such as cataract extraction or a glaucoma filtration procedure.

If each postoperative cataract patient were carefully examined, nearly all would show some degree of choroidal detachment.[34] On occasion the detachment becomes acutely severe if a wound leak develops, and the patient at that point notices sudden loss of vision. These symptoms, coupled with a large elevation in the posterior pole, may suggest retinal detachment, but careful examination reveals that the elevation is more solid in appearance and that the ora serrata can easily be visualized without scleral depression (Figs. 9-16 and 9-17). This latter finding is a definite tip-off that the detachment is choroidal rather than retinal.

Choroidal detachment may also result from surgery for a retinal detachment and is often due to choroidal hemorrhage from the subretinal fluid drainage site. Such detachments may occur at the time of surgery or may not become apparent until 24 to 48 hours later.

Choroidal Effusion Syndrome

In 1963 Schepens and Brockhurst described a form of nonrhegmatogenous retinal detachment which was noted in the fifth and sixth decades of life.[26] At

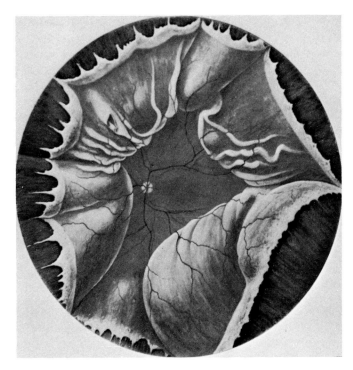

FIG. 9-16. Schematic representation of overlying retinal detachment. Note horseshoe tear at ten o'clock. (Courtesy of Dr. CL Schepens and Retina Foundation, Boston, Mass)

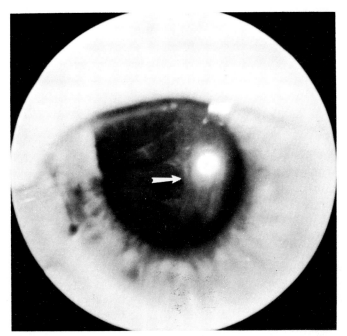

FIG. 9-17. Choroidal detachment, showing the ora serrata (*arrow*) in the middle of the pupil.

first these were mistaken for rhegmatogenous retinal detachments with small breaks, but when they universally did poorly with surgery the syndrome of choroidal effusion was recognized and described. Findings include choroidal detachment in association with the nonrhegmatogenous retinal detachment and an increase in cerebrospinal fluid protein. Both males and females are affected by the disease. Treatment at present consists of the administration of steroids. Bullous central serous chorioretinopathy may also cause shifting subretinal fluid, and must also be differentiated from rhegmatogenous retinal detachment.

Traumatic Choroidal Detachment

Blunt trauma is an uncommon cause of choroidal detachment, but may in rare instances precipitate its occurrence. Usually the blow is severe, and there are often additional findings such as dislocation of the lens and hyphema.

Penetration of the sclera and choroid by a missile or an instrument heralds a severe ocular injury which may be accompanied by hemorrhagic choroidal detachment.

Differential Diagnosis

The major conditions from which choroidal detachment must be differentiated are (1) rhegmatogenous retinal detachment, discussed earlier in this chapter, (2) primary intraocular tumor (most often choroidal melanoma; see Chap. 7), (3) choroidal hemangioma (discussed under differential diagnosis of malignant melanoma, in Chap. 7), (4) vitreous hemorrhage, and (5) metastatic tumor. Metastatic tumor (see Chap. 7) is usually not a problem in the differential diagnosis, since there may be a previous history of mastectomy or of lung or gastrointestinal tumors which could represent the primary lesion. In addition, metastatic tumors are likely to be multiple, and generally have a more sessile appearance than choroidal detachment. Choroidal detachment is also located more anteriorly than melanomas, metastatic tumors, or choroidal hemangiomas.

Hemorrhage into the vitreous is also not apt to cause a differential diagnostic problem. The red blood cells in the vitreous are easily seen on slit lamp biomicroscopy. If the hemorrhage is from a proliferative retinopathy such as diabetes, scleral depression often allows one to see the peripheral retina satisfactorily enough to rule out retinal or choroidal detachment. As the hemorrhage clears the periphery will become easier to see; the last portion of the fundus to become visible is the posterior pole.

By contrast, vitreous hemorrhage from a posterior vitreous detachment and retinal tear often is so massive that even with scleral depression the fundus periphery cannot be visualized. This is a clinically significant differential diagnostic finding and suggests the presence of a retinal tear. Complete bed rest with binocular patches and elevation of the head will usually allow the blood to settle in the retrohyaloid space within 24 to 48 hours. At this time, since the majority of retinal breaks occur above the horizontal meridian and especially superotemporally, a retinal tear, if present, may be identified and treated.

Diagnostic Aids

One clinical test that is frequently overlooked is transillumination. This may be easily done when the eye is anesthetized with topical anesthetic, and can differentiate a peripheral solid tumor, which does not transilluminate light, from a choroidal detachment, which does. However, occasionally hemorrhagic retinal detachments will not transilluminate well. Ultrasound can also be useful in differentiating a retinal detachment, which can frequently be traced back to the disc, from a choroidal detachment, which extends beyond the ora serrata. Finally, if a tumor is strongly suspected the ^{32}P test may be useful. All of these procedures are discussed in Chapter 2.

REFERENCES

1. **Benson WE, Grand MG, Okun, E:** Aphakic retinal detachment. Arch Ophthalmol 93:245–249, 1975
2. **Brockhurst RJ, Lam KW:** Uveal effusion, II. Arch Ophthalmol 90:399–401, 1973
3. **Byer NE:** Clinical study of retinal breaks. Trans Am Acad Ophthalmol Otolaryngol 71:461–473, 1967
4. **Byer NE:** Changes in and prognosis of lattice degeneration of the retina. Trans Am Acad Ophthalmol Otolaryngol 78:114–125, 1974
5. **Byer NE:** Prognosis of asymptomatic retinal breaks. Arch Ophthalmol 92:208–210, 1974
6. **Byer NE:** Prognosis of asymptomatic retinal breaks. In Strieff EB (ed): Modern Problems in Ophthalmology. New York, S Karger, 1974, pp 103–108
7. **Colyear BH, Pischel DK:** Clinical tears in the retina without detachment. Am J Ophthalmol 41:773–792, 1956
8. **Cox MS, Schepens CL, Freeman HM:** Retinal detachment due to ocular contusion. Arch Ophthalmol 76:678–685, 1966
9. **Custodis E:** Scleral buckling without excision and with Polyviol implant. In Schepens CL (ed): Importance of the Vitreous Body with Special Emphasis of Reoperations. St. Louis, Mosby, 1960, pp 175–182
10. **Davis MD:** The natural history of retinal breaks without detachment. Arch Ophthalmol 92:183–194, 1974
11. **Foos RY:** Zonular traction tufts of the peripheral retina in cadaver eyes. Arch Ophthalmol 82:620–632, 1969
12. **Foos RY:** Vitreoretinal juncture over retinal vessels. Albrecht von Graefes Arch Klin Ophthalmol 204:223–234, 1977
13. **Freeman HM:** Current management of the giant retinal breaks. In Pruett RC, Regan CDJ (eds): Retina Congress. New York, Appleton-Century-Crofts, 1972, pp 435–463
14. **Freeman HM:** The fellow eye in patients with giant tear. Trans Am Ophthalmol Soc 76:343–382, 1978
15. **Freeman HM, Schepens CL:** Innovations in technique for drainage of subretinal fluid: transillumination and choroidal diathermy. Trans Am Acad Ophthalmol Otolaryngol 78:829–836, 1974
16. **Freeman HM, Schepens CL, Humphrey WT, Elzeneiny IL, Moura R:** Transillumination and choroidal diathermy in the drainage of subretinal fluid. In Pruett RC, Regan CDJ (eds): Retina Congress. New York, Appleton-Century-Crofts, 1972, pp 391–396
17. **Gonin J:** Die Beziehungen der Retinalzystem zur Netzhautablosung. Klin Monatsbl Augenheilkd 67:316, 1921
18. **Gonin J:** Treatment of detached retina by searing the retinal tears. Arch Ophthalmol 4:621–625, 1930

19. **Hovland KR, Schepens CL, Freeman HM:** Developmental giant retinal tears associated with lens coloboma. Arch Ophthalmol 80:325–331, 1968

20. **Jaffe NS:** Complications of acute posterior vitreous detachment. Arch Ophthalmol 79:568–571, 1968.

21. **Jesberg DO, Schepens CL:** Retinal detachment associated with coloboma of the choroid. Arch Ophthalmol 65:163–173, 1961

22. **Lincoff HA, McLean JM, Nano H:** Cryosurgical treatment of retinal detachment. Trans Am Acad Ophthalmol Otolaryngol 68:412–432, 1964

23. **Linder B:** Acute posterior vitreous detachment and its retinal complications: a clinical biomicroscopic study. Acta Ophthalmol [Suppl] (Kbh) 87:1–108, 1966

24. **Michaelson IC, Stein R:** A study of the prevention of retinal detachment. Ann Ophthalmol 1:49–55, 1969

25. **Pemberton JW, Freeman HM, Schepens CL:** Familial retinal detachment and the Ehlers-Danlos syndrome. Arch Ophthalmol 76:817–824, 1966

26. **Schepens CL, Brockhurst, RJ:** Uveal effusion. I. Clinical picture. Arch Ophthalmol 70:189–201, 1963

27. **Schepens CL, Okamura ID, Brockhurst RJ:** The scleral buckling procedures. I. Surgical technique and management. Arch Ophthalmol 58:797–811, 1957

28. **Shafer DM:** Retinal detachment after phacoemulsification. Trans Am Acad Ophthalmol Otolaryngol 78:28–30, 1974

29. **Spencer LM, Foos RY:** Paravascular vitreoretinal attachments: role in retinal tears. Amsterdam, Exerpta Medica, International Congress Series No. 222:1527–1534, 1970

30. **Spencer LM, Foos RY:** Paravascular vitreoretinal attachments. Arch Ophthalmol 84:557–564, 1970

31. **Straatsma BR, Allen RA:** Lattice degeneration of the retina. Trans Am Acad Ophthalmol Otolaryngol 66:600–613, 1962

32. **Straatsma BR, Foos, RY, Krieger AE:** Rhegmatogenous detachment: pathogenesis, prophylaxis, and principles of management. In Duane TD (ed): Clinical Ophthalmology. New York, Harper & Row, 1976

33. **Stratford TP, Shafer DM:** In Schepens CL, Regan CDJ (eds): Controversial Aspects of the Management of Retinal Detachment. Boston, Little, Brown, 1965, p 51

34. **Swyers EM:** Choroidal detachment immediately following cataract extraction. Arch Ophthalmol 88:632–634, 1972

35. **Tasman W:** Posterior vitreous detachment and peripheral retinal breaks. Trans Am Acad Ophthalmol Otolaryngol 72:217–224, 1968

36. **Tasman W:** Peripheral retinal changes following blunt trauma. In Streiff ED (ed): Modern Problems in Ophthalmology. New York, S. Karger, 1974, pp 446–450

37. **Verdaguer TJ, Rojas B, Lechuga M:** Genetical studies in nontraumatic retinal dialyses. In Streiff EB (ed): Modern Problems in Ophthalmology. New York, S Karger, 1975, pp 35–39

38. **Weidenthal DR, Schepens CL:** Peripheral fundus changes associated with ocular contusion. Am J Ophthalmol 62:465–477, 1966

39. **Winslow R, Tasman W:** Juvenile retinal detachment. Most common cause in children Trans Am Acad Ophthalmol Otolaryngol 85:607–618, 1978

Index

Numerals in italics indicate a figure; t in italics following a page number indicates a table.